Special Issue

Suicide: Individual, Cultural, International Perspectives

Antoon A. Leenaars, PhD, Ronald W. Maris, PhD, and Yoshitomo Takahashi, MD, Editors

Special Issue, Suicide and Life-Threatening Behavior, 27(1), Spring 1997
Guilford Publications, New York
1997

Published by The Guilford Press
A Division of Guilford Publications
72 Spring Street, New York, NY 10012

This volume was published simultaneously as *Suicide and Life Threatening Behavior*, Volume 27, Number 1, Spring 1997

ISBN 1-57230-240-2

Last digit is print number: 9 8 7 6 5 4 3 2 1

Printed in the United States of America

SUICIDE: INDIVIDUAL, CULTURAL, INTERNATIONAL PERSPECTIVES

Editors

Antoon A. Leenaars
Ronald W. Maris
Yoshitomo Takahashi

Preface

The 29th annual conference of the American Association of Suicidology (AAS) was entitled Suicide: Individual, Cultural, International Perspectives. The senior editor, then President of AAS, set the theme and invited the keynote speakers. The event proved to be "the ideal place for the fruitful exchange of important thoughts and fresh concepts" (Shneidman, 1996). It was "a bountiful intellectual feast" (Shneidman, 1996). The manuscripts in this volume are the core keynote papers of that feast, somewhat augmented to add to the Gestalt of the menu. In this way, we hope to share this cultural/global event.

The purpose of the conference, and thus of the volume, is quite simple: understanding the individual within her or his cultural/global world. To say any more of the purpose would simply be redundant. Our mission, of course, is enhancing the effectiveness of suicide prevention in America and across the world.

The papers in this volume embrace both clinical introspective accounts and general objective reports. This resonates to Windelband's (1904) division of the possible approaches to knowledge between the *nomothetic* and the *idiographic*. The tabular, statistical, arithmetic, and demographic nomothetic approach deals with generalizations, whereas the idiographic approach involves the intense study of individuals – the clinical methods, history, and biography. In this latter approach personal documents are frequently utilized: personal documents such as case material, therapy notes, test data, letters, logs, memoirs, diaries, autobiographies, suicide notes. Let us, before addressing the topic at hand, explore the views on the idiographic approach in more detail; the other – the nomothetic approach – is well engrained in mental health studies and science in general.

Allport (1942) has provided us with a classical statement on the advantages of an idiographic approach. Allport (1962) notes that psychology is "committed to increasing man's understanding of man," men in general and man in the particular. What concerns psychology deeply is individual human personality. John Stuart Mill, in fact, had proposed that we make such a distinction in science, both being critical, although some scientists object strongly to the study of individual cases.

Allport (1962) provides the following:

> Suppose we take John, a lad of 12 years, and suppose his family background is poor; his father was a criminal; his mother rejected him; his neighborhood is marginal. Suppose that 70 percent of the boys having a similar background become criminals. Does this mean that John himself has a 70 percent chance of delinquency?

Allport answers:

> Not at all. John is a unique being. (p. 411)

Yet, we would add that John also lives in a unique cultural neighborhood (world). Allport (1962), in fact, noted that the real concern about the idiographic and nomothetic is developing methods that are more rich, flexible, and precise, that "do justice to the fascinating individuality" of each individual. Runyan (1982, 1983) has more recently outlined a detailed defense for idiographic approaches. Our volume is in the idiographic tradition and at the same time in the more widely accepted nomothetic tradition. Science would be overly limited without either (Leenaars, DeLeo, Diekstra, Goldney, Kelleher, Lester, & Nordstrom, 1997). Let's begin with the individual perspectives.

Part I examines the unique suicidal mind. It consists of four conference presentations (plus one addition): a discussion of adolescent suicide in a cultural perspective; a suicide of a young adult whose unique cultural background may have contributed to this death; a presentation of an adult case, highlighting culture and ego-ideal; and an overview of suicide in an older adult, highlighting our changing times.

If one accepts the importance of the individual, a number of issues emerge. We fundamentally believe that "no man is an island unto himself." Thus, although it may seem paradoxical, we asked Ronald Maris to speak on social suicide (the addition). This, we believe, is not only necessary but a legitimate avenue to understanding the person in his or her world. We need to not be narrow-minded in understanding the individual.

The individual – such as John – is among other things a social being. Individuals live in a meaningful world. Culture may well give us meaning in the world. It may well give the world its theories/perspectives. This is true about suicidology. Western theories of suicide, as one quickly learns from a cultural perspective, may not be shared. Suicide has different meanings for different cultures. Shneidman (1985) cautions us, when making "cross-cultural comparisons, do not make the error of assuming that a suicide is a suicide" (p. 203). This is as true about the United States as it is about other nations. America is, in fact, an area of cultural diversity. Part II explores this diversity of meaning by examining the following five topics on American peoples: an overview of suicide in various Americans; a discussion of suicide as the scourge of Native American people; a review of the cultural paradox of suicide among African Americans; a comparison of Caucasian and Asian groups, a presentation of a San Francisco study; and a discussion of current knowledge of Mexican Americans, making suggestions for the direction for research that has implications for all cultures in America.

Yet, we believe that we must go beyond the United States and explore suicide across the world to accurately answer the questions "Why do people kill themselves?" and "Why did that individual kill himself or herself?" Indeed, as we head towards the year 2000, it is clear that we live in a global world. This is true for economics, politics, literature, and suicidology. To be unaware of the international perspective would result in one's understanding of the individual being overly barren and misleading. However, our need is not simply factual but also emotional as, for example, we join in the grief of the 16 victims of the kindergarten class and the survivors of the suicide in Dunblane, Scotland, in March of 1996. None of us can forget the horror of that suicide – and we dedicate this volume to the victims and survivors of that disaster. Often the individual's rage against herself or himself is also rage against the world. In that sense, we are all survivors of the suicides across the world. Part III presents four manuscripts: An overview of suicide across the globe, highlighting the importance of personal meaning of suicide; a discussion of suicide in Canada, noting the differences and similarities between Canada and the United States; a perspective on suicide in Europe with special reference to a unique study of attempted suicide; and a reflection on culture and suicide in Japan.

By way of background, the following introduces our contributors in order of appearances in the text:

- **Alan L. Berman**, PhD, ABPP is Executive Director and a Past President of the American Association of Suicidology (AAS), and in private practice at the Washington (DC) Psychological Center, PC. He is the lead author of *Adolescent Suicide: Assessment and Intervention* and editor/coeditor of four suicidology books.
- **Antoon A. Leenaars**, PhD, CPsych, is a faculty member at the University of Leiden, the Netherlands, and in private practice, Windsor, Canada. He was the first Past President of the Canadian Association of Suicide Prevention (CASP) and is a Past President of AAS. He has published 10 books in suicidology and is the Editor-in-Chief of *Archives of Suicide Research*, the official journal of the International Academy for Suicide Research (IASR).
- **John T. Maltsberger**, MD, is a Lecturer

in Psychiatry at Harvard Medical School and a member of the faculty of the Boston Psychoanalytic Institute. He is a Past President and a Dublin Award winner of the AAS. He has published numerous books in suicidology including, as coeditor, *Treatment of Suicidal People.*

- **Joseph Richman**, PhD, is in private practice in New York and Professor Emeritus at Albert Einstein College of Medicine. He is a Past Board Member and Dublin Award winner of the AAS and a world expert in gerentological suicidology. He has published numerous books in the field including, as coeditor, *Suicide and the older adult.*
- **Ronald W. Maris**, PhD, is Professor of Sociology and Psychiatry at the University of South Carolina, Columbia. He is a Past President and a Dublin Award winner of the AAS, and outgoing Editor-in-Chief of *Suicide and Life-Threatening Behavior*, the official journal of the AAS. He has published numerous books, including, as the lead coeditor, *Assessment and Prediction of Suicide.*
- **David Lester**, PhD, is Executive Director for the Study of Suicide in Blackwood, New Jersey, and Professor at Stockton State College, Pomona. He is a Past President of the International Association for Suicide Prevention (IASP) and a cofounder of IASR. Focusing primarily on suicide and homicide, he has published over 50 books, including, as coeditor, *Suicide and the Unconscious.*
- **Marlene EchoHawk**, PhD, is a respected Native American psychologist and Deputy Chief of Alcoholism and Substance Abuse, Department of Health and Human Services, Albuquerque, New Mexico. She has worked diversely to address suicide among the Native American and Alaskan Native people, especially youth. She has presented – and published – many papers in suicidology including the keynote address at the 29th annual conference of AAS printed in this volume.
- **Jewelle Taylor Gibbs**, MSW, PhD, is the Zellerback Family Fund Professor in Social Policy, Community Change and Practice, School of Social Welfare, University of California at Berkely. In 1987 she received the McCormick Award from the AAS for her contribution to research on minority youth suicide. An expert on African Americans and minorities, she has published numerous volumes including, as author, *Race and Justice: Rodney King and O. J. Simpson in a House Divided.*
- **Julia Shiang**, PhD, is Assistant Professor at Pacific Graduate School of Psychology and Stanford University School of Medicine, Palo Alto, California. As an expert on Asian Americans, she has published extensively in the areas of suicidology, acculturation, and culture. **Robert Blinn**, PhD, is a clinician at Nebraska Mental Health Center and in private practice in Lincoln, Nebraska. **Bruce Bongar**, PhD, is Professor at Pacific Graduate School of Psychology and Stanford University School of Medicine. **Alan Schatzberg**, MD, is Chair of the Department of Psychiatry at Behavioral Services at Stanford University School of Medicine. **Boyd Stephens,** MD, is Chief Medical Examiner, and **Donna Allison**, PhD, is Statistician and Data Analyst, both at the Medical Examiner's Office, San Francisco.
- **Joseph D. Hovey**, MA, is a doctoral candidate in clinical psychology at the University of Michigan, Ann Arbor. An emerging expert on Latino-Americans, his research interests include suicide and acculturation. **Cheryl A. King**, PhD, is a faculty member at the Departments of Psychiatry and Psychology, University of Michigan. Having published extensively in adolescent depression and suicide risk, she is President-Elect of AAS.
- **Isaac Sakinofsky**, MD, is a faculty member in psychiatry, University of Toronto, and Director of the Department for Suicidology Research at the Clarke Institute of Psychiatry. Having received the first Research Award of CASP for his noted Canadian research in the field of suicide and its prevention, he was an

early Board Member of CASP, hosting CASP's first regional conference. He has published extensively including, as coeditor, *Suicide in Canada.*

- **Armin Schmidtke**, PhD, is a faculty member at the Psychiatric Clinic, University of Würzburg, Germany, and Secretary of IASR. He is a principal investigator at the WHO/Euro Multicentre Study of Parasuicide, being recognized for his expertise in suicide and attempted suicide. He has published extensively including, as coeditor, *Attempted Suicide in Europe.*
- **Yoshitomo Takahashi**, MD, is Deputy Chief, Department of Psychopathology, Tokyo Institute of Psychiatry, and a Board Member of the Japanese Association for Suicide Prevention. Recognized internationally as an expert in suicidology, he hosted the first conference on suicidology in Japan. Having published extensively in the field, he edited *Life and Death from a Psychiatric Perspective* (in English and Japanese).

These people are scholars from the United States and from across the world. Although no volume can present the complexity of the individual and cultural diversity in America and the world, we believe that the authors in this issue have something important to say on the topic. We hope that the reader agrees as she or he gains understanding of the suicidal individual in his or her cultural/global world.

Antoon A. Leenaars, PhD
University of Leiden

Ronald W. Maris, PhD
University of South Carolina

Yoshitomo Takahashi, MD
Tokyo Institute Of Psychiatry

REFERENCES

Allport, G. (1942). *The use of personal documents in psychological sciences.* New York: Social Science Research Council.

Allport, G. (1962). The general and the unique in psychological sciences. *Journal of Personality, 30,* 405–422.

Leenaars, A., DeLeo, D., Diekstra, R., Goldney, R., Kelleher, M., Lester, D., & Nordstrom, P. (1997, in press). Consultations for research in suicidology. *Archives of Suicide Research, 3.*

Runyan, W. (1982). In defense of the case study method. *American Journal of Orthopsychiatry, 52,* 440–446.

Runyan, W. (1983). Idiographic goals and methods in the study of lives. *Journal of Personality, 51,* 413–432.

Shneidman, E. (1985). *Definition of Suicide.* New York: Wiley.

Shneidman, E. (1996, April). Letter on Twenty-ninth annual conference of the American Association of Suicidology, St. Louis.

Windelband, W. (1904). *Geschichte und Naturwissenchaft* (3rd ed.). Strassberg: Hertz.

PART I. Individual Perspectives

1
The Adolescent: The Individual in Cultural Perspective

Alan L. Berman, PhD

Case vignettes are presented to highlight the idiosyncratic dynamics and special cultural influences that describe adolescent suicides. Extrapolated from these cases are a series of aphorisms about the study of adolescent suicide and about adolescence, meant to inform both clinicians and researchers on the need to better attend to the individual in context of his or her cultural influences.

CASE VIGNETTES

Ali.

The first thing one noticed was Ali's blank stare. It was a Haldol stare; 10 mg., q.i.d.

The medication was working. He was in control; or, more honestly, the medication was. In the hospital, before the medication was prescribed, he had broken a window and attacked his fellow patients. Now he had been released in care of his father, who, just the day before, had flown in from Libya to take him home.

At 19 Ali was to go into the army, but he didn't want to. So he decided to leave his home and come to the United States to study. He was not a good student. In Libya he had concentrated on weight lifting. He claimed he was "third [best] in his country." Now he had to prove himself in an academic arena. He had to take his high school equivalency test in order to apply for entrance to the university. But he had failed, by "only four points, on [his] second try," he said.

He felt shamed and humiliated. He faced returning to his family as a failure; and once again – the press of military service. These he could not tolerate. He broke.

He called it "a great pain in my head." No, not voices, but an unbearable ache. Shneidman (1993) would call it *psychache*, but Ali knew only that, in his country, "to put out the pain in [one's] head," [you] "put fire to the head." That's how the police found him, on Main Street, his hair ablaze. Next stops: the State Hospital, Haldol, and an ignominious return home in the care of his family.

In Ali's culture, this was not a suicide attempt. In Ali's culture, this was not even viewed as a self-destructive act. Nor was this a psychotic behavior, as his doctors at the State Hospital believed. In Ali's culture, the burning of one's hair was a means of exorcism, culturally prescribed. We are reminded that behavior is not culture-free. We are reminded to understand the individual within the cloak of his or her identity.

I wish to present to you a series of brief case vignettes to highlight our understanding of the suicidal adolescent within the context of his or her culture. I present these cases to you as a psychologist, trained to have deep respect for the need to better understand the individual. Each case speaks uniquely to this theme; each reminds us of the idiosyncracies of suicide. Each case, with its individual dynamics and special cultural influences, reminds us that there is no typical suicidal adolescent.

In the Shoshone culture, family cohesion is important. Western Shoshone families were nomadic. They lived off the land, harvesting and hunting, as needed, in small family bands in a seasonal pattern of life. Poorly equipped to stem the tide of western expeditions of White settlers who

Alan L. Berman is Executive Director of the American Association of Suicidology and with Washington Psychological Center, PC, Suite 602, 4201 Connecticut Ave., N.W., Washington, DC 20008.

rapidly depleted traditional food supplies, western Shoshone families soon came under government control and, in 1863, signed a treaty agreeing to settle on reservations.

Reservation life stripped the Shoshone of their nomadic culture. It also greatly challenged the traditional extended family culture. For example, tribal governance on the reservation required cooperation among families, but tribal elections created a hierarchy among families—those with and those without power. One family having authority over another was not to be tolerated, so anarchy, rather than self-government, ruled.

In the same vein, excessive individualism was not tolerated. The concept of self-advancement and individual success, in contrast to working *for the family*, was antithetical to the Shoshone culture. In consequence, for example, a rancher who made a profit on the sale of livestock was expected to either share his success with his siblings and cousins or to diminish himself in some way. Depression, alcohol, and/or often drugs served as vehicles for self-attack. Suicide was the ultimate expression of unacceptable success.

For the student, educational achievement posed a paradox. The successful student had to leave the reservation to advance, to go to boarding school or college. But this was a violation of the norm, for the family was left behind. If you left, you "copped out." Most teens who were bright enough to leave returned, having dropped out of school, often only months before graduation. Those who graduated also returned to live in a normatively depressed culture that could not support or give expression to their individual competencies. The few college graduates were as likely to be employed as maintenance workers at the reservation hospital as they were to be unemployed.

Clay.

Clay had just turned 20. Years earlier, he had left boarding school to return home to live with his parents; his father was a chronic alcoholic. At 2:00 a.m., after a night of drinking, Clay walked into the reservations's Law and Order Office, brandishing a gun and threatening to shoot himself. The officer on duty, a second cousin, tried to give him reason not to but to no avail. The bullet perforated his bowel. At the hospital they performed a temporary colostomy and referred him to Mental Health. "I don't need anyone," he yelled; then he denied being angry at anyone but himself. He said he was bored, that he "had nothing to do at home except see his brother and sister."

Three years before, at the age of 17, Clay had been arrested for being intoxicated and, with rifle in hand, threatening to kill himself. Just last year, at 19, he had ingested "about 14 large white pills" and was hospitalized overnight. At that time Clay told Mental Health that he had no intention of doing this again. The social worker wrote in his chart, "I feel he is sincere."

Seven months after his last suicide attempt Clay would be dead—an overdose while intoxicated.

Betty.

Betty was only 14, the youngest of five. Her parents had divorced when she was very young. Her mother died just last year of alcohol-related causes; she was 28. Betty now lived with her father, her uncle, her grandfather, and her brothers. Like Cinderella, she was responsible for cooking and cleaning. She was not permitted to complain. Depressed over her mother's death, frustrated and angry at her family life, she became her mother. She stayed out all night drinking. Having neglected her assignments and too hungover to go to school, she chose truancy and sleep during the day. Yelled at by her family, she responded by overdosing twice and stabbing herself in the abdomen, all within six months.

Culture is the nutrient medium within which the organism is cultivated. Suicidality grows, as well, when that culture is pathological. Family pathologies are notable for being suicidogenic. They spawn children at risk. Sometimes, when that risk is acted out, suicidal behavior functions to remove the adolescent from the pathogenic family. Suicidal behavior can be designed to protect, to rescue the self from an otherwise certain annihilation.

Suicidal behaviors may serve to remove the adolescent to places and people that are intended to provide sanctuary. We in position to help like to believe that we create holding environments, wombs of safety and security that foster a healing process. This is the culture of the helping environment, repairing and nurturing. Sometimes, however, even these cultures fail. Sometimes they are suicidogenic.

Alicia.

Alicia was only 13, a sixth grader of mixed Indian and Hispanic heritage. This was her first and only psychiatric admission, a remarkable fact given her family history. Her mother reportedly was murdered when Alicia was but one or two years old. She steadfastly believed that her biological father was the murderer.

As a young child, she went to live with relatives in South America. They abused her physically. She returned to the United States and, from the ages of five to eleven, lived with her father and three older brothers. Her father and a brother, allegedly, abused her sexually. She told a schoolteacher about her abuse and was removed from her home by the Department of Youth and Family Services. Charges were placed against her father and her brother.

Her first foster home placement did not work out, but she was growing attached to her current foster parents. Concurrently, she feared being rejected; she knew this would happen if she got too close to them. When she learned that she would be expected to testify against her father and brother, she got depressed and preoccupied. Over several months, she reported difficulty sleeping at night, experiencing recurring flashbacks of her abuse, difficulty concentrating – with failing school grades, and thoughts of dying by taking poison or putting a sweater around her neck to choke herself. One time she scratched her wrist with a razor blade, "to let out the pain." She got admitted to the hospital.

She was comorbidly diagnosed: major depressive disorder, single episode; dysthymic disorder; and posttraumatic stress disorder. She was medicated with antidepressants. When she showed signs of hypomania – including silliness, giggling, and sexually inappropriate remarks – she was treated with lithium carbonate and chlorpromazine. She was evaluated medically and neurologically. She was multiply therapized: individual therapy, group therapy, recreation therapy, art therapy, and occupational therapy. She was put on suicide precautions. During the first month of hospitalization, she spoke of hanging herself with a bedsheet or towel. She planned to use a metal wire brought to her by a fellow patient. As long as she expressed suicidal thoughts and wishes, she was kept on closely observed status. She told a nurse, "I've always thought of killing myself since the day I was born. . . . I know I'll commit suicide some day, it's just too much pressure." She was frequently asked by staff about suicidal feelings, intentions, and plans. She consistently indicated to staff that she would come to them before she would do anything to hurt herself. She signed a contract agreeing to tell staff if she felt like harming herself. This apparently made the staff more comfortable.

During this hospitalization, she and her foster parents grew more distant. Finally, three months after her admission, they severed their relationship. Over time, as she showed some signs of improvement, she was removed from the constant observation to frequent observation and then to frequent awareness status – this in spite of signs that her mood and behavior were unpredictable and recent notice from the court that she would soon be called to testify about her father and brother's abuse.

She began to discuss and consider discharge dispositions with staff members. She interviewed for a group-living facility, but was rejected. She was given a second chance and was excited in anticipation of a repeat evaluation. In therapy, she rehearsed her interview style. She was eager for discharge. She told a peer, "I might be leaving soon." The attending psychiatrist noted that her mood was labile, but she wanted to maintain her status in order to enhance her shot at being accepted by this placement facility.

Two weeks after her first interview, Alicia got her second chance. She did poorly. Returning to the ward, she was sullen, rude, and demanding. She blamed the facility's doctor for not accepting her. She literally clung to her only friend in the hospital, who was about to be discharged. She angrily shouted at another patient to stop staring at her. Her medical chart noted she had "a horrible day."

By the next day, she was commenting that she didn't care about the outpatient facility. The attending psychiatrist noted that "she didn't express strong feelings about being rejected." Her mood and behavior were described in the charts as "softer, less complaining, claiming not to be sad." Someone else noted in her chart that she was "stiff and guarded" with staff. With her peers she was observed to be both "social and playful." She denied suicidal intent or ideation. There was no change in the status of observation. After all, her contact was still in effect.

The next day was Sunday. She was awakened at 9:15 a.m. and was noted to be dawdling in her room. The nurse encouraged her to prepare for breakfast. She said, "I'm going to the bathroom."

At 9:30, the nursing staff noted a knotted sheet over her closed bathroom door. On opening the door, Alicia fell to the floor. She was warm to the touch but blue, not breathing, and pulseless. CPR was initiated and a code was called, but she could not be resuscitated. Five minutes later she was pronounced dead.

The assessment of acute risk in an adolescent at chronic risk for suicide requires clinical judgment. During the days before Alicia's suicide, she recapitulated all the events that had precipitated her admission to this hospital. Hers was a culture of rejection, abandonment, and loss. The rejection and abandonment by her foster parents, the rejection by her potential and desired discharge placement, the refusal to accept the upcoming discharge (loss) of her friend, and the anticipatory trauma and stress of her upcoming court appearance all should have signaled increased watchfulness. Moreover, Alicia's rapid shift of mood the day before her suicide should have been another red flag. In a context of woundedness, you simply don't expect the calm she expressed. We provide no true sanctuary to our patients if we fail to observe, assess, and use clinical judgment at times of transitional stress. When a suicide contract, agreed to by a patient devoid of trustability, is assumed by caretakers to be trustable, we have participated in providing that patient a culture of poor care.

John.

Same hospital; same psychiatric unit; four months earlier, only three weeks before Alicia was to be admitted: John was 14, a high school freshman. Maybe someone should have wondered why it had been two days since he scratched his wrists that his parents brought him into the emergency room. Maybe they were jaded by the fact that this was his third low-lethality suicidal behavior. One year previously he had begun outpatient psychotherapy after overdosing on about a dozen acetiminophen. Only a month ago he made his first attempt to scratch his wrists. That prompted a psychiatric evaluation and the initiation of antidepressant medication.

This attempt followed an arrest when he and a friend were caught by the police on the roof of a neighbor's house. He was charged with breaking and entering, trespassing, and resisting arrest. He was released to the care of his mother. She later, in family interview at the hospital, minimized the significance of his suicidality. "He's just manipulative," she said.

In the emergency room, however, he told the liaison psychiatrist that he did not want to live. He threatened to obtain a gun, spoke of intense anger toward his mother, and reported both sleep and appetite disturbance. He also talked openly of obsessional thoughts and compulsive behaviors. He claimed to wash his hands and feet up to 12 times a day. "This is where sins collect," he claimed; like Christ, he "was washing away his sins."

He was admitted on suicide precautions to the psychiatry service with diagnoses of major depression, recurrent, severe and obsessive–compulsive personality disorder with schizotypal features. The attending psychiatrist entered an order to change his antidepressant medication from Paxil to Zoloft, and to increase dosage from 50 to 100 mg, but the nurse failed to transcribe the order on the Medication Administration Record. No one detected her omission.

On the unit John still talked of purchasing a handgun. His initial ward behavior was noted as silly and noncompliant, often testing of staff. His mental status evaluation documented inappropriate affect and thought content dominated by death wishes. Family medical history revealed a history of bipolar disorder, a ten-year history of depression in his mother, and a maternal uncle's suicide. The index attempt was documented as his fourth since childhood, the first at age 4 when he jumped out of an upper-story bedroom window.

A family meeting on the second day of his admission documented marital stress. In addition, his parents minimized John's pathology and pressed for early discharge. They were specifically asked not to discuss discharge with him independent of staff involvement or until given permission by the attending psychiatrist. By the third day John's status was reduced to frequent awareness, in spite of chart notations regarding continued inappropriate smiling and a complaint by a female patient that John had put his hand down her pants.

John's continued denial of suicide intent led to a discontinuance of all precautions on day four, even though he spent two 15-minute periods in a quiet room for oppositional behavior and for throwing ice cream during lunch.

On day five he refused to participate in a community meeting. His unit behavior was described as intrusive and attention seeking. Early that afternoon he met with his parents and sister. After that meeting he told the head nurse that his "mother said [he's] better" and that they had agreed he'd be discharged in two days. His affect was notably brightened. Two hours later he was found on the floor of his room hanging by a bedsheet. He was cyanotic and apneic. CPR and the efforts of a code team failed to resuscitate him.

THE APHORISMS

What I wish to extrapolate from these cases are some aphorisms, some simple truths that might serve to inform us as we get to better know our individual adolescent patients. In order to accomplish this I must digress briefly and provide some personal history. This is a sort of confession. You see, my interest in adolescence and the route I took to become a psychologist have the same roots, both stumbled upon (or over) quite by accident.

In my junior year of college, quite broke and needing a part-time job, I fortuitously came across a notice posted on a bulletin board outside the Department of Social Relations. "Advanced Undergraduate Needed to Assist Professor on Large Federal Research Grant," it said, speaking only to me.

Fancying myself an "advanced undergraduate," I snatched the notice from its moorings, entered the Soc-Rel office, and boldly announced that their search was over. To keep this reasonably brief, I was hired by an Associate Professor named Edward McDill. Mac, as he insisted he be called, had just arrived at Hopkins to work along with Jim Coleman. As some of you may remember, Jim Coleman was, by then, "the foremost mathematical sociologist of his age" (Moynihan, 1995), having gained fame for his landmark and heretical report "Equality of Educational Opportunity." This study documented that student achievement and aspirations were influenced more by social status and peer relations than the quality of the school one attended. Mac, in Coleman's wake, had secured a large, several-year Health, Education, and Welfare (HEW–the predecessor to DHHS) grant to further this work and study the student cultures of high schools and their influences on academic achievement and intellectualism.

This was going to be a tough assignment. I was to be a general all-around Man Friday to Mac and several of his graduate students. As a group of six, I being the only undergraduate, we traveled around the country to a number of American public coeducational high schools to administer extensive questionnaires to what totaled to 20,000 students, in addition to their teachers and their parents.

With training, my job was to proctor the classroom administration of these surveys, code the questionnaire responses, and key-punch them to cards for computer analyses (a truly useless skill in the 1990s). In addition, I was to chauffer this merry band of six to about half of their data collection sites and to drink merrily with them each night on the road (a truly useful skill for an "advanced undergraduate").

I was taught some more useful skills also. Mac insisted I learn how to program (in a now-dead language call Fortran) and to use a computer; in those days it filled an entire library room. I also was taught how to draw sociograms and to interpret "marginals," so I could participate in the data analyses that took through my senior year. In order to free me from class so that I could leave Baltimore and travel with the research team, Mac arranged to develop and mentor an Independent Study course or two along the way. He made me read about research and discuss my understandings with him; he introduced me to Coleman's *The Adolescent Society* (1961) and C. Wayne Gordon's *The Social System of the High School* (1957).

So, by my senior year in college, I had a fair amount of experience in large-scale research and, in particular, the study of the adolescent and the adolescent culture. At the age of 21, I was beginning to understand how to make it in high school! I have no doubt that these experiences and Mac's support and encouragement to stay in social science (not to minimize the value of his recommendation) abetted my admission to graduate school and initiated my career. I also know that these early experiences gave me deep respect for research, the understanding of the individual, and for placing that understanding within the context of the individual's culture.

With that autobiographical digression, I can return to my thesis.

Aphorism 1: In spite of many sightings, to date, science has failed to prove the existence of adolescence.

Science begins with an operational definition of its subject. Try, if you will, to define the period of adolescence. We might well enough agree that it begins with puberty—demarcated by physiological changes we can measure. But even this parameter must be gender specific, as girls tend to reach puberty about two years ahead of boys; and dynamic, as the age of onset of puberty has been decreasing over the past several decades. And when does adolescence end? Typically, the end of adolescence is thought to coincide with sociocultural life transitions, for example, movement away from family and mastery of the practical demands of independent living. In Western societies, adulthood is thought to begin in one's early 20s (Levinson, Darrow, Klein, Levinson, & McKee, 1978). But more and more of today's young adults live at home under the protective wing of their parents, and the average age of first marriage keeps increasing. Thus the end of adolescence yet needs to be defined. As with God, we must still prove the existence of adolescence.

Moreover, I suggest that we borrow from the lexicon of our colleagues in geriatrics and recognize that adolescence, if we are truly to learn about it, needs to be subdivided into periods or stages akin to "young-young," that is, puberty to the beginning of "old-young," that is, from then to whenever we define the beginning of young adulthood.

Take note that even our federal governments maintain this muddle, suggesting through our oft-quoted statistics that adolescence extends from the age of 15 to 24. Who among you would argue that a 15-year-old should be grouped with a 24-year-old in the same data set analysis?

With regard to suicide, these age differences are important in that suicidal behaviors are not static through the years of adolescence. Indeed, onset curves for the age of first suicide attempt are progressive, with rates increasing for each subsequent age group after puberty (Lewinsohn, Rohde, & Seeley, 1996). Suicide attempt rates at ages 14–15 are more than double those at ages 12–13 (Lewinsohn et al., 1996). Similarly, rates of suicide ideation do not increase linearly through the teen years (Lewinsohn et al., 1996). Lastly, completed suicide rates in the United States for 20- to 24-year-olds are more than a third greater than those for 15- to 19-year-olds; yet the rates for 15- to 19-year-olds are increasing at a faster rate than those for the older group. We simply must begin to differentially study these youngsters.

Aphorism 2: G. Stanley Hall was right in comparing adolescents to lower primates.

The word *adolescence* is derived from a Latin root meaning "to grow up." The avenues toward maturity travel in many directions; are differentially paved; and may twist, turn, and confuse, as readily as they transport the child toward adulthood. We've not yet well described the better roads to take.

G. Stanley Hall, as you know, was the founder of the first American research laboratory in psychology (at Hopkins) and the first president of the American Psychological Association. Writing almost a century ago, Hall (1904) said that adolescence prepares youth for "higher and more completely human traits" (p. xiii). The avenues he suggested in order to socialize children involved allowing them to first play as savages, then as barbarians and nomadic wanderers. Hall was a Darwinian and he appreciated the need for acculturation.

My point here is that we need a fresh understanding of those cultural influences that (1) move the nomadic child toward a healthy maturity versus those that (2) move the wanderer on a pathway toward a premature death by suicide.

As but one example of the former, we are only beginning to spend our meager research dollars on the study of protective factors, those cultural influences that buffer the child from becoming suicidal. Results of this work are essential to inform more modern generations of prevention and treatment programs, to emphasize the development of life and social skills (i.e., wellness enhancement) over programs that are pathology focused (e.g., deficit reduction models).

As but one example of the latter, we yet know painfully little about what cultural forces influence the adolescent who has once made an early-age suicide attempt to never again be suicidal—even though he or she is now appropriately marked as forever at risk—in contrast to what influences an attempter to repeat an attempt or to ultimately complete suicide. What are the familial, peer, and therapeutic influences that differentially define the life or death pathways of those once suicidal?

Aphorism 3: G. Stanley Hall was wrong. Adolescence should not be delayed until the youngster is mature enough to handle it.

If you recall, it was Hall (1904) who applied the phrase "Sturm und Drang" to the period of adolescence. Hall's model was one of stress and turmoil, instability and distress. A brief glance at indices of dysfunction during the adolescent years suggests that today's youth face greater threats and destabilizing influences than did prior generations. For example:

- In the United States, rates of divorce and the consequent numbers of children living in single parent households continue to rise (Office of Educational Research and Improvement, 1991).
- Cohort studies of depression have found that depressive syndromes occur at higher prevalence and have a younger age of onset today than for earlier generations of adolescents (Leon, Klerman, & Wichmaratne, 1993).
- The number of 14- to 17-year-olds arrested for serious crimes continues to be unacceptably high.
- Births to unmarried women aged 15–19 were more than 50% higher in the late 1980s than in the mid-1970s and 140% greater than they were when I was 17 (Office of Educational Research and Improvement, 1991).

And I should not have to cite this year's statistics on HIV seropositivity or drug usage to make this point.

Most profoundly, our statistics on adolescent suicide suggest that now, more than ever before, Hall's characterization of this period is apt and fitting. Given the high rates of completed suicide and the prevalence of attendant psychopathologies, such as substance abuse, it is indeed tempting to agree that, if possible, we should declare a moratorium on adolescence until adolescents have the maturity to weather its storms.

But wait; there is yet another perspective on today's adolescents (Office of Educational Research and Improvement, 1991).

- Less than 2% of children under 18 were involved in divorce last year, and there has been no significant change in rates of divorce in the United States since the mid-1970s.
- The number of births per 1000 teenage women age 15–17 is less than it was in the early 1970s.
- And the number of arrests per 1000 14- to 17-year-olds in the United States in the late 1980s was less than what it was a decade earlier.

These are trends that ought to spark some optimism among those of us who projected doom and gloom in the late '70s as we extrapolated the projected increase in the size of the adolescent population toward the century's end.

Moreover, occasional suicide ideation appears to be common to adolescence, with perhaps as many as 60% of teens identifying having a transient suicidal thought. This suggests that the modal adolescent thinks about suicide; yet only a small proportion of adolescents act on that thought and less than 2% report making a serious suicide attempt in any one year (Centers for Disease Control, 1994). It is suggested here that many adolescents may bend under the pressure during these years of turmoil, but only a small fraction of them break.

As it is painfully evident that those adolescents whom we need to better observe and help are a small subset of the adolescent population as a whole (e.g., those with psychopathology), it should be equally obvious that we are yet at some distance from being able to discriminate adolescents in high-risk groups who are those more, versus less, likely to act on suicidal urges. For example, Shaffer and Bacon (1989) have noted that the ratio of depressed teenagers to depressed teenage suicides is approximately 660:1. Clearly, we still need to encourage research that distinguishes those few depressed adolescents who do make suicide attempts from those many depressed adolescents who do not. It should concern us greatly that not one of the teen cases presented earlier was seen to be *at risk at the time of their suicidal behaviors.* This was true in spite of all of them displaying serious signs of risk, including depression. If we are failing to assess risk in those who provide us direct and blatant cues, how can we hope to better detect those whose signs are less observable?

This leads me to my last aphorism and to what my early dalliance with sociology taught me.

Aphorism 4: Adolescence is not a culture-free developmental period.

I have become identified among my peers as a passionate defender of the individual case study. Indeed, I feel passionate about the need for clinicians to figuratively and carefully peel the onionskins from those individual patients who present to us for help. But, I must remind you that no individual exists in a vacuum, especially our adolescents.

Adolescence is truly demarcated by a relative progression from the culture of the family, to that of the peer system, to that of one's own making (e.g., marriage and family). Inherent in these systems linking the individual to his or her culture are personal needs for belonging, affiliation, and succorance, to name but a few (cf. Shneidman, 1993).

Adolescent suicide is mostly an interpersonal event. Nonfatal attempts are almost universally instrumental behaviors designed to change or influence the adolescent's relationship with another person. The overwhelming majority of triggering events for suicidal behaviors in adolescence are interpersonal: from conflicts with parents to rejections in peer relationships.

From the family culture to the peer culture, the social system within which the adolescent struggles for a sense of acceptance, approval, and status contributes mightily to the stresses that strain a fault line into an earthquake.

Coleman (1961) and McDill referred to these cultural influences as "climate effects." Their hypotheses predicted that in every social context, certain types of behavior were socially rewarded, and that the dominant motivation of the adolescent was to achieve and maintain a general social status within the social system. Conformity to the norms of the majority group was the goal, because this produced acceptance, and this pertained even when these norms were defined around a theme of deviance from the larger culture: cultists have norms, punks have norms, skinheads have norms, etc. It is reasonable, therefore, to predict that suicidal behaviors are triggered when there is a social threat – that is, a real, perceived, or anticipated loss of acceptance; or a perceived inability to maintain, or attain, a desired status; or when the immediate cultural influence is suicidogenic, such as we see when we have a cluster of suicide attempts within a deviant group of teens.

Let's briefly return to the cases I presented earlier and examine how these climate effects interacted with individual pathologies to produce the observed suicidal behaviors.

- Ali, the 19-year-old Libyan student, felt shamed and humiliated, and feared returning to his family as a failure. He lacked status at home and in his desired autonomous life.
- Clay, the 20-year-old Shoshonean, was unable to free himself from a culturally prescribed life of alcohol and boredom. He lived in a suicidogenic culture with

very high suicide rates that maintained a mental health system that did not take suicidality seriously.

- Betty, the 14-year-old from the same reservation, having lost her mother to alcohol, became her mother; she rejected the family that used and neglected her, turning to alcohol and suicidal behavior in protest. She, too, lived in Clay's culture and was attempting to achieve status by identifying with her mother.
- Alicia, the 13-year-old abused female was also desperate for a family. She killed herself when she was not accepted into a group-living facility. The hospital staff showed no increased concern for her suicidality in response to her latest rejection. Incredibly, they seemed unaware of the import of this event given her dynamics and history. She was desperate for status and belongingness in a family.
- John, the 14-year-old who killed himself in the same hospital, had intense conflict with his mother, who consistently minimized the seriousness of his suicidality. His suicide immediately followed a family visit during which his mother told him he was better and would be discharged soon from the hospital. This occurred in spite of her being told by hospital staff not to discuss discharge; yet the staff allowed an unsupervised visit between John and his parents to occur. The importance of this family to John's suicidality was simply not understood by his caregivers.

We can do little to prevent the triggering precipitants to suicidal events; yet we can do much to increase our awareness of individual and idiosyncratic vulnerabilities to them. This awareness allows us to buffer or preventively intervene specific to the cultural influences on any one patient. If we understand well enough the need for the individual to feel valued by and important to others, and attend to the individual in these contexts, suicidal behaviors – even among the mentally disordered – have less likelihood of occurring. This marriage between psychological and sociological awarenesses lies at the heart of good clinical care.

Ann Beattie, the novelist, wrote eloquently of this awareness when she penned the following about raising children in her book *Picturing Will* (1989). I close with this excerpt as a humble reminder to both parents and clinicians of the daunting task we assume in attempting to hold on to this essential awareness as we attempt to care for our children and bring them through a healthy adolescence:

> Insist on eye contact when you speak. Do not let others turn the child upside down. Check the babysitter's references. Lock the cabinet that contains the cleaning products below the sink. Regular visits to the doctor. Two security blankets, so one can be washed. Check toe room in shoes regularly, by depressing the leather underneath your thumb. Comb tangled hair from the ends up. Speak out against environmental hazards. Look out for danger, but do not communicate your fear to the child. Buckle your seat belt. Cut down on consumption of red meat. Learn a jingle called "The Toothbrush Is Your Friend." Advise him not to bother kitty when she's eating. Try to make a game of gathering up toys with the child. Don't overdramatize the scary parts of books. Do everything right, all the time, and the child will prosper. It's simple as that, except for fate, luck, heredity, chance, the astrological sign under which the child is born, his order of birth, his first encounter with evil, the girl who jilts him in spite of his excellent qualities, the war that is being fought when he is a young man, the drugs he may try once or too many times, the friends he makes, how he scores on tests, how well he endures kidding about his shortcomings, how ambitious he becomes, how far he falls behind, circumstantial evidence, ironic perspective, danger when it is least expected, difficulty triumphing over circumstance, people with hidden agendas, and animals with rabies.

REFERENCES

Beattie, A. (1989). *Picturing Will.* New York: Random House.

Centers for Disease Control and Prevention. (1994). Health-risk behaviors among person 12–21 years – U.S., 1992. *Morbidity and Mortality Weekly Report, 43*(8), 129–132.

Coleman, J. S. (1961). *The adolescent society.* New York: Free Press of Glencoe.

Gordon, C. W. (1957). *The social system of the high school.* Glencoe, IL: Free Press.

Hall, G. S. (1904). *Adolescence.* New York: Appleton.

Leon, A. C., Klerman, G. L., & Wickmaratne, P. (1993). Continuing female predominance in depressive illness. *American Journal of Public Health, 83,* 754–757.

Levinson, D. J., Darrow, C. N., Klein, E. B., Levinson, M. H., & McKee, B. (1978). *The seasons of a man's life.* New York: Knopf.

Lewinsohn, P. M., Rohde, P., & Seeley, J. R. (1996). Adolescent suicide ideation and attempts: Prevalence, risk factors, and clinical implications. *Clinical Psychology: Science and Practice, 3*(1), 25–46.

Moynihan, D. P. (1995, December 31). The lives they lived. *The New York Times,* Sect. 6, p. 25.

Office of Educational Research and Improvement, U.S. Department of Education. (1991). *Youth indicators 1991: Trends in the well-being of American youth.* Washington, DC: U.S. Government Printing Office.

Shaffer, D., & Bacon K. (1989). A critical review of preventive intervention efforts in suicide, with particular reference to youth suicide. In Alcohol, Drug Abuse, and Mental Health Administration, *Report of the Secretary's Task Force on youth suicide. Volume 3: Prevention and interventions in youth suicide* (pp. 23–30) (DHHS Publ. No. ADM 89-1623). Washington, DC: U.S. Government Printing Office.

Shneidman, E. S. (1993). *Suicide as psychache.* Northvale, NJ: Jason Aronson.

2
Rick: A Suicide of a Young Adult

Antoon A. Leenaars, PhD

A small but concerning percentage of completed suicides are seen as having left no clues. The classical case, albeit a literary one, is Robinson's *Richard Cory.* These people often dissemble, even about their suicide risk. An even smaller group of these individuals present themselves in therapy without communicating a sign of suicide risk. Utilizing an idiographic approach, the case of a young adult male (Rick) is presented. The narrative reconstruction gives voice behind the man's mask. The autopsy reveals a young man who was in deep pain and unable to adjust to life's demands. Rick lacked ego strength, being overly narcissistic and having deeply troubled, symbiotic attachments to his family in a world of interpersonal isolation. In the end, even the help of his therapist, who tried to reach through the mask, was not enough and Rick killed himself. The pain had become unbearable. A few guiding remarks for such cases are offered, noting that therapists must constantly address the dissembling in some suicidal patients.

"Suicide happens without warning." This is a myth that Shneidman challenged around 1952 and incorporated into a number of publications (e.g., Shneidman & Mandelkorn, 1970). He stated that in fact, "Studies reveal that the suicidal person gives many clues and warnings regarding suicidal intentions." Another fact, according to Shneidman, is that "Of 10 persons who kill themselves, 8 have given definite warnings of their suicidal intentions." However, is it really a fable that "suicide happens without warning"?

Studies by McIntosh, Hubbard, and Santos (1983) and Leenaars, Balance, Pellarin, Aversano, Magli, and Wenckstern (1988) supported the belief that people believe that "suicide happens without warning" is a myth. Yet, clinically, the concern is this: if 8 out of 10 people give warnings, what about the other 2? Goldblatt (1992) and Litman (1995) have separately noted that a small but important percentage of completed suicides are seen as having left no clues. A minority of these people are most perplexing to even the most veteran suicidologist. How do we understand and predict their suicide?

The classical case, albeit a literary one, is Robinson's *Richard Cory* (1953). The poem describes Richard Cory as a "gentleman from sole to crown." He was "human," "rich," "favored," and "schooled"; and, in fact, people "thought that he was everything." Then, as the poem ends:

> And Richard Cory, one calm summer night,
> Went home and put a bullet through his head. (p. 38)

That suicide happened without warning. The Richard Cory type of patient is, in fact, a person whom many of us experience in our clinical career. Bongar and Greaney (1994), in their studies, have found that the odds are greater than 50% that a psychiatrist, and greater than 20% that a psychologist will lose a patient to suicide over the course of his or her career. A patient committing suicide is, thus, not a rare event, although the Richard Cory patients do not comprise all of them. The fact is that over 80% of the patients who killed themselves did leave clues. The

---

Antoon A. Leenaars is with the University of Leiden and in private practice, Windsor, Canada. Address correspondence to the author at 880 Ouellette, Suite 806, Windsor, ON N9A 1C7 Canada. Fax: 1-519-253-8486

There is nothing more important in our clinical practice with suicidal patients than sound consultation. I am pleased to acknowledge the unequaled clinical consultations of John T. Maltsberger, Joseph Richman, and Susanne Wenckstern regarding this case.

other 20% raise our anxiety, with the Richard Cory type being even more infrequent. I here discuss such a patient who did not give a warning before his death, in the hope of understanding the Richard Cory type patient better.

RECONSIDERATION OF CLUES

Shneidman (1994) has recently reconsidered his perspective on clues to suicide. He asked "How it is that some people who are on the verge of suicide . . . can hide or mask their secretly held intentions?" Shneidman suggests that many clues are veiled, clouded, and guarded, some even misleading. He argues that there are individuals who live secret lives. These people do not communicate. On the Rorschach, as an example for clinicians, they would score a high Lambda (Exner, 1986). These people do not process and/or mediate the stimuli in the usual way, having a defensive intent to avoid the situation. Often this reflects a basic coping style, with conscious and unconscious elements in the process (Leenaars & Lester, 1996). Shneidman calls it *dissembling.* To dissemble means to conceal one's motives. It is to disguise or conceal one's feelings, intention, or even suicide risk. These people wear "masks." Most clinicians encounter such people, not only suicidal patients. Shneidman (1994) stated:

> We suicidologists who deal with potentially suicidal people must . . . understand that in the ambivalent flow and flux of life, some desperately suicidal people . . . can dissemble and hide their true lethal feelings from the world. (p. 395)

I believe that this is especially true with our adolescents, and perhaps even more with young adult patients. These young people often dissemble with their parents, girl/boyfriend, therapist, everyone.

Young Adulthood

Young adulthood is a discrete time line in development (Frager & Fadiman, 1984; Kimmel, 1974). It has its unique biological, psychological, cultural, and sociological issues. I tentatively support the position in limiting this time line from 18 to 25 (Kimmel, 1974; Neugarten, Moore, & Lowe, 1965). Of course, no developmental period can be rigidly defined chronologically, and at best the 18-to-25 range approximates what can only be defined developmentally; that is, some people mature earlier, others later than the mean.

Adolescence is a stage marked by the development of a sense of identity. The young adult continues to develop this sense of identity, evolving a finer and more discrete sense of who he/she is in relation to others. Not distinct from this process, the demand to master the challenge of intimacy emerges as the central issue of young adulthood. Erikson (1963, 1980) was one of the first to pioneer work on intimacy (intimacy vs. isolation) in young adulthood, noting that one must have a sense of who one is before on can appreciate the uniqueness of another. Although the capacity to relate to others emerges earlier, "the individual does not become capable of a fully intimate relationship until the identity crisis is fairly well resolved" (Kimmel, 1974, p. 23). Often, before such development, the individual can only avoid genuine closeness or engage in narcissistic relationships. As Frager and Fadiman (1984) note:

> Without a sense of intimacy and commitment, one may become isolated and be unable to sustain intimate relationships. If one's sense of identity is weak and threatened by intimacy, the individual may turn away from or attack whatever encroaches. (p. 152)

I would add, even oneself!

Research on suicide in Young Adults

Research regarding any psychological area of young adulthood is scarce (Kimmel, 1974). Studies on suicide in this group are even scarcer. Even the volumes on suicide that are apparently directed to include this age group (e.g., Klerman, 1986) disappoint us, for they only take note of our lack of knowledge about this group of individuals. Insights are often generated from general developmental issues, but we do not find specific information about suicide (see Levinson, 1986). Often young adults are classed together with adolescents, a taxonomic maneuver both theoretically and empirically unsound. There have been exceptions to the overlapping taxonomy in the field (e.g., Leenaars, 1989, 1991; Rickgarn, 1994); however, clearer definitions are needed in the research of young adults, which needs to be integrated into life span perspectives (Leenaars, 1991). Thus, the clinician working with young adults is cautioned about using current research, needing to be clear and distinct about age, cultural issues, and more in clinical applications.

Idiographic Approach

Case studies have an important place in suicidological history (Allport, 1942; Shneidman, 1985). Despite some controversy about the admissibility of the idiographic approach, I present here a clinical case of a Richard Cory type patient that I was able to reconstruct through a psychological autopsy. I do not address treatment, only the psychological understanding of an individual. I primarily provide the material from the therapist's notes, with other data as needed from the autopsy.

THE CASE

Intake

Rick was a 23-year-old male who first arrived at the office of the therapist quite distraught. He was agitated, perturbed. The therapist asked, "What is wrong?" Rick reported that he had been charged with sexually harassing suggestions to an unknown female. He was primarily focused on the arrest, fearing conviction and jail.

He reported that the charge was upsetting him, presenting initially only permutations of that crisis. He denied other problems. However, further inquiry revealed that he had experienced a rejection by a girlfriend, Sally, about two years earlier. They had dated for two years, planning to marry. However, one evening, when he went out with some friends despite Sally's objections, he learned that Sally had had an affair with one of his few friends. She broke off the relationship. Rick had not dated since the breakup. Having found the unknown female attractive, he had made suggestive remarks to her. When asked about the harassment, he admitted that he had been making such remarks for a few years, and earlier before dating Sally. He reported that he had never been charged, questioning the therapist about possible consequences.

Rick's mood was depressed, exhibiting a markedly diminished interest. There was no weight loss although he complained about insomnia. He was agitated and exhibited mild problems in concentrating. When asked about suicide ideation or any attempts, he denied any suicidal intent. However, he did reveal that his mother's brother had killed himself many years earlier. Rick identified his parents as problematic for him, suggesting a stressful history at home. He admitted to use of steroids (which, according to records, were not used subsequent to the arrest).

With regard to his history, Rick had no previous mental health history; he denied any disturbances or treatments. However, he did report that he believed that his mother was disturbed (although he was initially vague about what he meant). Rick's medical history was unremarkable. He had the usual childhood illnesses. Rick's parents, both of British ancestry, met at high school and had been married for 28 years. Rick described their relationship as empty, stating "they never talk." Rick's father was in sales, often being away from home. His mother had never been employed outside the home. Rick had one sister, Susan. Susan was one year older, having married at 17. He did report, however, that his mother was too involved in her life, much like his own.

Rick's personal history, according to him, was generally unremarkable. He was an average student. He reported no problems at school, completing grade 12. He did, however, suggest that problems increased after school. He became more isolated, primarily associating with one good friend, David. He reported only one female relationship in the past, that is, Sally.

The Process

Utilizing a time sequence format, let me outline the complexity of the case as it is recorded in the treatment notes:

When asked about his reason for seeing the psychologist, Rick stated "the charge." He reported that he had been told to see a psychologist by the arresting officer. Fearing jail, he followed the suggestion. The therapist noted that there was likely no personal motivation, only being propelled by the crisis.

The records indicate that he attended five sessions, missing a number of appointments. The missed appointments were explained as forgotten. Rich had discussed, upon inquiry, his ambivalence about seeing the therapist. He expressed that it made him anxious although jail was anticipated to be worse. Of note is the fact that Rick was anxious about everything. Avoidance was a general pattern. He talked about deep shyness. For example, going to grade 9 had been a devastating event. He simply withdrew, becoming very isolated in his first year of high school.

The anxiety and ambivalence further hindered the treatment. Rick often lacked focus, asking the therapist to focus. The notes often raise questions about dissembling. The therapist also noted that the first "no show" occurred after receiving a letter from the therapist for his lawyer. Rick had requested the letter to assist in the pending trial. The content of the letter reflects Rick's ambiguity to treatment but clearly states the need.

A number of aspects of Rick's life were learned.

Sally had been his best friend. The relationship was "everything." It was his first and only sexual relationship, and he described the sex as binding. They were always together. One night, his friend David asked him to go drinking. Despite Sally's request not to go, he went. He then discovered that Sally met with one of his other friends that night, engaging in sex. That was the end of the relationship.

He described the event as painful, building an even higher "wall" around him. He had mentally collapsed although he denied any suicidal reaction. He stated that he had met other women but "always found something wrong with them." He remained alone, insulating himself from other relationships. The therapist noted that Rick associated the current symptoms to that trauma (and more). Of critical note was Rick's relationship to his mother. She was described as an adult child of an alcoholic, having been herself prone to alcohol abuse.

His mother was overly obsessive, often negative. A diagnosis of depression is likely. She was described as critical and overly controlling, exhibiting extreme panic reactions if things were not her way. He stated "Everything had to be right." For example, if he arrived home 10 minutes late, she panicked. As another example, if one moved any of her over 100 Royal Dalton figurines, she would rage mercilessly. The family life, in fact, revolved around her wants, following what he called "strict British rules." The family, according to Rick's report, was dysfunctional. His mother controlled his sister and father and him, instilling guilt in everyone. It is, in fact, the guilt induction that is relevant to his verbal harassment; after the statements, he would be very harsh and self-critical.

The harassment was likely related to a cycle of depression, describing boredom before making such statements. He would fear the female and then be excited by the sexual nature, only to subsequently self-punish himself. It was suspected that at a deeper level the harassment was related to his anger towards his mother. Of note is the fact that Rick admitted that he knew that he would get caught, suggesting that he often did things knowing that he would be punished.

The last session of the first series of visits involved discussing his dysfunctional family. Rick and the therapist focused not only on his mother but his father. His father, the son of British immigrants, was described as very passive, following his wife's wishes. The father often spent the little time that he had at home cleaning the house because Rick's mother wanted it "spotless."

Rick returned to the therapist after 6 months without a scheduled appointment. He was extremely upset, having just returned from court, where he had been found guilty. Rick was not jailed but the judge had ordered Rick to seek treatment as a condition of parole.

When Rick returned for a scheduled appointment, he indicated that he had to be there, still lacking self-motivation. Rick's parole officer contacted the therapist from time to time. The issue of participation was figural; "no shows" were frequent. There were a number of hiatuses in the contact. He attended 17 sessions every other week, which met the parole condition. Yet, the notes are full of questions about his lack of communication and openness. The therapist asked from time to time about termination; Rick continued to state that he had to attend. Obviously, such situations are not optimal and one would question whether there even was a therapeutic alliance.

When Rick first returned, he reported that he was dating Gloria, who was a friend from his high school years. Gloria and Rick quickly bonded. Rick described the sex as more mutual than with Sally. He now described the former relationship as negative, always having to make the advances. He stated that he was now "always happy." However, at home, his problems remained.

The discussion in subsequent sessions focused on his relationships such as with Sally, describing her as controlling and castrating. He now also saw his harassing statement as his way to control women. He associated those insights to his mother. Yet, his relationship with Gloria was different, stating "I don't want to be ____ whipped." Rick often associated these discussions to insecurity, not only his, but that of men in general. That was especially true about his father, someone with whom he identified. That identification was likely deeply problematic for Rick. Discussion occurred about his mother's narcissism, much like Sally's. However, insight into his own narcissism was lacking. He reported to the therapist that he needed a mask, "a false self" to cope, suggesting that his mother would not accept him otherwise. Obviously, as the therapist noted, "the not being able to move the figurines in the house" issue was only the conscious tip of the iceberg.

According to Rick, he needed to avoid and dissemble. He stated that it allowed him to cope with his mother. He described, for example, his mother's confrontation about Sally, "Did you have a good ____?" Although Rick held that the question was inappropriate, he felt guilt. Again, the therapist associated these guilt inductions to his own criminal charge.

Equally, Rick associated his mother's sexual inquisitiveness to his parents' marital problems. He reported that they did not sleep together. He questioned the relation, suggesting divorce would have been best, including for him and his sister.

After a few months, a long hiatus occurred in therapy. Upon Rick's return, the therapist noted that the defenses were stronger. The walls were often there, with only a few specific breaks occurring. On one occasion, the therapist noted: "Rick talks. That is unusual." Rick, in fact, reported that no one talked in his family, stating that it is "the British" way. "No one speaks", he said. The anger towards his passive father was especially noted, and the therapist and Rick identified a circular system. They discussed that Rick's father's passivity actually reinforced the rage of his mother. Rick concluded that it caused a lot of pain, as did Sally and the harassment, describing it all as "hopeless."

The father's role, subsequently, became figural. Rick reported that he never talked to his father; even worse, he "never went to a ballgame, nothing." That too was described as painful. Much later, Rick revealed that his father had been an abused child, having been removed at the age of 8 from his home by the child protection agency. His father's relationship to his family of origin ceased to exist; he never saw his siblings. Despite those insights, Rick deeply lacked a closeness to his father and that lack was critical.

The notes in the next few months suggested that the relationship to Gloria was developing. One issue that emerged, however, was Rick's lack of openness. Rick reported that Gloria "wants more discussion." However, there was even greater dissembling. Rick never invited Gloria to his home; indeed, the parents subsequently revealed that they never knew that she even existed. Yet, Rick felt positive, talking about a future. Rick saw Gloria increasingly as his only attachment. More and more he saw his mother – and Sally – as negative. He explored issues of marriage and children. Their sexual relationship was discussed equally positive, describing it as "more healthy" than with Sally.

Gloria was accepting of Rick, whereas his relationship to other women was not. His mother especially was not so. He once stated "Nothing is okay." He suggested, however, that his mother acts like the victim, that she blames him, his sister, and her husband for everything. Only with Gloria did he describe a closeness. He noted that being in therapy allowed him to be more open, being so different from at home. One time he stated if his mother communicates, "she'll say it through the door."

In the last few months, Rick's attendance was more sporadic, attending only once per month. The therapist noted that Rick went on vacation, traveling with his friend David. Of particular notice about that relationship was David's relationship to his own girlfriend. Rick described them as opposite, not talking. He described David's girlfriend like his mother, wanting very little sex. There were a lot of issues, yet David married her. Rick's reaction was one of fear, asking "Is that what happens?" Of course, the association to his parents is obvious.

The records indicate that the crime was only figural when the parole officer contacted the therapist. There were no subsequent charges and Rick denied any involvement in harassment. However, the issue was always associated to acute anxiety and some relapse prevention work is documented in the treatment.

During Rick's penultimate visit, the therapist noted that Rick's defensiveness increased. They spoke about his motivation for treatment. Rick stated, "it is a parole condition as needed." His parole officer continued to ask about his attendance. However, parole would cease in six months. The therapist noted: "So, he'll be here till the end of parole."

Rick did, however, reveal new consequences to his charge. He had always wanted to be a police officer, and Rick learned that option was now closed, a painful recognition. Indeed, Rick expressed anger at the charge, the lawyer, the system.

During his last visit, Rick reported that he was doing well (dissembling?). He focused only on his relationship to Gloria. They had gone out for lunch and she had told him that she loved him, but he questioned his love. Indeed, he stated that his parents did not love each other, asking if anyone did. Rick was especially intellectual in the discussion about relationships, citing that David's was a failure too. He asked questions like "What is love?" and "Is there love?" Most important, he asked if he was capable of love. Rick was especially and unusually inquisitive about the therapist's thoughts. What did he think love was? Did the therapist love? Did he think people did? At the end of the session, Rick reflected on a movie about a mother's love for her son. It was, of course, something that he wanted; yet it was something that he never felt.

The next appointment was not kept. The therapist was called by Rick's sister, who announced that Rick had "passed away" of a heart attack (familial dissembling?). Later, the therapist learned that Rick had killed himself.

PREDICTION AND ASSESSMENT

Could Rick's suicide have been predicted? Suicide is generally difficult to predict and assess. Recently, in response to awareness of the inherent difficulties in predicting suicide, the National Institute of Mental Health (NIMH) of the United States (Garrison, Lewinsohn, Marsteller, Langhinrichsen, & Lann, 1991) reviewed all available assessment instruments used to study suicidal behavior and concluded: *Few, if any, are useful.* Despite this state of affairs, the NIMH group did isolate two instruments, designed for populations across the life span, that have some potential in predicting suicide risk (i.e., the intent to kill oneself). They are: (1) *Beck Suicide Intent Scale* (BSIS) and (2) *Lethality of Suicide Attempt Rating Scale* (LSARS). Would these tests have assisted in predicting Rick's risk? Both of these instruments would, I believe, have resulted in a low score for Rick. Indeed, it is unlikely that a test will allow us to predict a Richard Cory type suicide. Most assessment is based on some direct or indirect clue, and when people dissemble, there is no such clue.

Probably the best approach to assessing risk with patients is the simple question "During the last 24 hours, what were the chances of you actually killing yourself: absent, low, moderate, high, very high?" Rick's records indicate that the therapist approached the issue twice with Rick. At intake, the therapist asked the question, but suicide intent was denied. There was no reported ideation and no plan, only that the mother's brother had killed himself (although that itself is, of course, a risk factor). The question arose on one other occasion. The therapist explored suicidal risk during the session when the mask came off ("Rick talked. That is unusual"). Rick had discussed feeling depressed and "hopeless." The hopelessness was about the loss of Sally; he still denied any suicide risk.

Understanding Suicide

If one attempts to understand suicide, one becomes aware over time of its enormous complexity. Suicide is not a psychopathological entity in the *Diagnostic and Statistical Manual of Mental Disorders* (DSM-IV–American Psychiatric Association, 1994). It is not merely a reaction toward external stress, although a recent traumatic downhill course (e.g., drop in income, a change in work, disgrace at work or office, separation and divorce) can often be identified. Rather, suicide is best defined as an event with biological (including biochemical), psychological, interpersonal, situational, sociological, cultural, and philosophical/existential components (Leenaars, 1996).

In understanding suicide risk in people, we need to be aware of behaviors that are potentially predictive of suicide. However, there is no such definitive behavior. Two concepts that have been found to be essential and helpful are *lethality* and *perturbation* (Shneidman, 1985). Lethality refers to the probability of a person killing him/herself, and on quantification scales ranges from low to moderate to high. It is a psychological state of mind. Perturbation refers to subjective distress (disturbed, agitated, sane–insane, decomposed) and can also be rated from low to moderate to high. Both have to be evaluated. It is important to note that one can be perturbed and not suicidal. Lethality kills, not perturbation.

With these two concepts in mind, suicide is, I believe, best seen as a multidetermined event (Leenaars, 1996). It is, metaphorically speaking, an intrapsychic drama on an interpersonal stage. From a psychological view, Rick, I believe, can be clinically understood from the following concepts, but not exclusively from these.

Intrapsychic

Unbearable Psychological Pain. The common stimulus in suicide is unendurable psychological pain. The person feels the pain of feeling pain, a psychache (Shneidman, 1985, 1993). Although, as Menninger (1938) noted, other motives (elements, wishes) are evident, the person primarily wants to flee from pain. The person may feel any number of emotions such as boxed in, rejected, deprived, forlorn, distressed, and especially hopeless and helpless. The suicide, thus, as Murray (1967) noted, is functional because it abolishes the painful tension for the individual; it provides relief from intolerable suffering.

Rick's life was full of pain. Despite his dissembling, he clearly felt pain. He was distressed, depressed, and boxed in. Yet there is no suggestion that it was unbearable. He did describe the situation at home as hopeless, but not as bottomless. The trauma with Sally was equally catastrophic; yet he escaped from that by his harassment. One wonders what became unbearable. In all probability, it was likely that the relationship to Gloria had failed. Was he again rejected? Or did he terminate the relationship? Did he believe that he could not love?

Cognitive Constriction. The common cognitive state in suicide is mental constriction, that is, rigidity in thinking, narrowing of focus, tunnel vision (Shneidman, 1985). The person is figuratively intoxicated or drugged by the constriction, exhibiting at the moment before the death only permutations and combinations of a trauma (e.g., imprisonment, poor health, rejection by a lover). In the suicidal mind, a possible solution becomes *the* solution.

Rick was constantly constricted. His vocabulary was full of words like "always" and "never." He was intoxicated with the loss of Sally, even two years later. Again, however, there is no suggestion in the records that suicide had been *the* solution, until he killed himself. Be that as it may, he had a propensity towards mental and psychological blindness.

Indirect Expressions. Complications, ambivalence, redirected aggression, unconscious implications, and related indirect phenomena are often evident in suicide. The suicidal person is ambivalent. The person experiences humility, submission, devotion, subordination, flagellation, and sometimes even masochism. Yet there is much more. What the person is consciously aware of is only a fragment of the suicidal mind (Leenaars, 1993). The driving force may well be unconscious processes (Freud, 1917/1974a; Leenaars, 1993; Leenaars & Lester, 1996).

Rick was deeply ambivalent towards his mother, Sally, maybe even Gloria. His harassments were redirected aggression; he was deeply angry at Sally and his mother. Submission, subordination, and flagellation were evident. Yet there was more. At a deeper level, there were painful attachments to Sally and his mother, and a yearning for a father who was psychologically absent. Indeed, I suspect that the unconscious processes in our dissembling patients are more important than the conscious ones.

Inability to Adjust. People with all types of problems, pain, losses, etc., are at risk for suicide. Although the majority of suicides may not fit best into any specific nosological classification, depressive disorders, manic–depressive disorders, anxiety disorders, schizophrenic disorders, panic disorders, borderline disorders, psychopathic disorders, and others have been related to some suicides (Leenaars, 1988; Sullivan, 1962, 1964). Depression may well be the most frequent disorder (Lester, 1992); however, suicidal people more frequently experience unbearable pain, not depression. Indeed, suicidal people see themselves as unable to adjust. Their state of mind is incompatible with accurate discernment of what is going on. Considering themselves too weak to overcome their problems, they do not survive life's difficulties.

Rick was depressed. His mood/behavior and verbal expression reflected that state of mind. He felt dejected, being hesitant in social contacts. He often isolated himself; in fact, his sexual harassments can be seen as primitive forms of seeking-out contact. There were obsessive–compulsive features and, thus, an identification with his mother. Rick also had some narcissistic features, something Goldblatt (1992) had associated to the Richard Cory type suicide.

Ego. The suicidal person's ego, the part of the mind that reacts to reality and has a sense of individuality, is a critical aspect in the suicidal act. Suicidal people frequently exhibit a relative weakness in their capacity to develop constructive tendencies and to overcome their personal difficulties (Zilboorg, 1936). The person's ego has likely been weakened by a steady toll of traumatic life events (e.g., loss, rejection, abuse, failure). A weakened ego correlates positively with suicide risk (Leenaars, 1988).

Rick lacked ego strength. Ego strength is a protective factor against suicide. He had experienced a steady toll of rejections; even the charge resulted in a loss of a dream, becoming a police officer.

Interpersonal

Interpersonal Relations. The suicidal person has problems in establishing or maintaining relationships (object relations). There frequently is a disturbed, unbearable interpersonal situation. Suicide appears to be related to unsatisfied or frustrated attachment needs, although other more intrapsychic needs may be equally evident, for example, achievement, autonomy, dominance, honor. Suicide is committed because of the thwarted or unfulfilled needs, needs that are often frustrated interpersonally.

Rick's object relations were problematic. The relationship to Sally was a calamity, resulting in self-destructive behavior (i.e., the harassment). Equally, his family was dysfunctional. There was insufficient individuality, being controlled by his mother. Such symbiotic relations, in fact, occur frequently in suicidal people. The system was inflexible, lacking open communication. Rick's needs, especially attachment, were frustrated. Yet, the relationship to Gloria was seen as a possible way to go on. But on his last visit, he confessed that he could not love.

Rejection–Aggression. The rejection–aggression hypothesis was first documented by Stekel in the famous 1910 meeting of the Psychoanalytic Society in Freud's home in Vienna (Friedman, 1910/1967). Loss is central to suicide; it is, in fact, often a rejection that is experienced as an abandonment. It is an unbearable narcissistic injury, an injury that leads to hate directed towards others and self-blame (Shneidman & Farberow, 1957). The suicidal person is deeply ambivalent and, within the context of this ambivalence, suicide may become the turning back upon oneself of murderous impulses (wishes, needs). Suicide may be veiled aggression—it may be murder in the 180th degree.

Rick felt rejected. Loss was related to his pain; it is likely that the rejection by Sally was a narcissistic injury. That fact makes it more probable that the loss of Gloria occurred. Be that as it may, much of Rick's pain was self-directed. He was deeply angry, even the harassment was aggressive.

Identification–Egression. Freud (1917/1974a, 1920/1974c) hypothesized that intense identification with a lost or rejecting person or, as Zilboorg (1936) showed, with any lost ideal (e.g., health, youth, career, freedom) is crucial in understanding the suicidal person. Identification is defined as an attachment (bond), based upon an important emotional tie with another person (object) (Freud 1921/1974d) or any ideal. If this emotional need is not met, the suicidal person experiences a deep pain (discomfort) and wants to egress, that is, to leave, to exit, to get out, to be dead.

Rick was deeply bonded to Sally and even more so to his mother. Those emotional ties were critical in Rick's behavior. His father, of course, was overly absent from his identification. Yet, the *essential* key to suicide, "I will kill myself," the egression, was not stated. Without this, lethality is difficult to evaluate. We did learn, subsequently, that the death was calculated to be discovered by his mother.

INTERPRETATION OF THE CASE

Thus, it can be concluded that theory is still a useful – if not the sole – avenue to understanding suicide, although even the best of suicidologists may have casualties. This is especially the case with patients that dissemble, such as Rick. Rick was highly perturbed at times; however, his lethality was low. Rick exhibited many of the outlined psychological commonalities of suicide; however, he equally lacked some of the key characteristics. None of our patients fit completely into our frames (Goffman, 1974).

Of importance is that Rick's profile fits, according to research, the characteristics of young adults who killed themselves. The suicide of young adults is most different from other adults across the adult life span (Leenaars, 1989). Although there may be other differences, Leenaars (1989) isolated critical differences in inability to adjust, ego, and interpersonal relations.

Even more than in other adults, suicide in young adults is related to their lack of ability to cope (Leenaars, 1989). They more often exhibit a psychological disorder. Rick was weakened and depressed. He exhibited a history of maladjustment. Not completely distinct from the inability to adjust, young adults are also more likely to exhibit a relative weakness in their capacity to develop constructive tendencies (Leenaars, 1989). They lack ego strength. Like all too many young adults, Rick did not overcome his personal difficulties. His ego, already at his young age, had been weakened by a steady toll of pain.

Consistent with theory (Erikson, 1963), however, the most important observation documented by Leenaars (1989) is that the suicide of young adults more than other adults is related to a disturbed, unbearable interpersonal situation. This is an observation of more or less, not presence or absence. Relationships are central in almost all suicides. However, it is especially with young adults that intimacy versus isolation is figural. It was for Rick. He had problems developing intimacy, even questioning if he could love. With rejection, especially from Sally, he isolated. He attempted to be intimate with Gloria but probably failed at the end. At home, he was isolated. He felt deeply alone. Maybe even his harassments were attempts at making connections. However, from his last session, one hears about a young adult painfully alone, much like his own father.

Thus, we can conclude that lack of attachment was an unbearable pain for Rick. Intimacy is the core conflict of young adults. A narcissistic injury likely occurred before his death. It would have added to the lethal mix of a lonely young man to allow him to jump into the abyss. Theoretically, it is known that such injury would have heightened the lethality.

To frame these observations more deeply, I would like to offer the following more general observations about suicide across the life span, not only in young adults:

Suicide is an intrapsychic and interpersonal event. However, the most significant unconscious processes in suicide may well be interpersonal (Leenaars, 1993; Maltsberger, 1986). This is, I believe, very true for suicide in young adults. Freud (1920/1974c) had already speculated on the latent interpretation that leads someone to kill him/herself: "probably no one finds the mental energy required to kill himself unless, in the first place, in doing so he is at the same time killing an object with whom he had identified himself and, in the second place, is turning against himself a death wish which had been directed against someone else" (p. 162).

People need to develop a strong identification with other people. Attachment, based upon an important emotional tie with another person, in a person's earliest development, was Freud's (1921/1974d) meaning for the term *identification.* The person (or other ideal) does not merely exist outside; rather, the object becomes introjected into one's own personality. Although the word *identification* has different meanings in the literature (see Hartmann, 1939; Meissner, 1981), I have here retained Freud's use of the term as *attachment.* Freud speculated:

> Identification is known to psychoanalysis as the earliest expression of an emotional tie with another person. . . . There are three sources of identification. First, identification is the original form of emotional ties with an object. Secondly, in a regressive way it becomes a substitute for a libidinal object tie, as it were by means of introjection of the object into the ego, and thirdly, it may arise with any new perception of a common quality shared with some other person who is not an object of the sexual instinct. (p. 105)

Freud's (1940/1974f) own use of the concept was divergent. In his later writings, he frequently used the concept of identification as a mechanism of structuralization, namely the superego. Although I am not suggesting that these views are not relevant, I wish to preserve *identification* to mean a deep primary attachment to significant people (e.g., parents) or some other ideal. Identification is a means of identifying with an object consciously and/or unconsciously, making it part of one's own internal world. It has a psychic existence in the mind.

Identification becomes a hallmark of one's early development. The attachment is deep within one's mind. The attachment is all too frequently symbiotic. As Litman (1967), noted, our "ego is made up in large part of identification" (p. 333). These identifications are associated primarily with one's parents, especially the primary caregiver. With loss, abandonment, excessive dependency, and other traumatic experiences in the relationships, especially if symbiotic, the attachment becomes dysfunctional. These identifications often get repeated in other significant relationships and the person experiences ongoing pain, becoming hopeless and helpless (Fenichel, 1954). This was true for Rick and was critical to his suicide.

Rick, of course, is not Richard Cory. Individuals are different. However, by the very fact that we are all human beings, there are commonalities. I have attempted to isolate some of these in the suicidal individual.

Shneidman (1994) wrote:

> If it is true that all the world's a stage, then some players, on occasion, may wear masks. And then, to paraphrase Melville – if man will help, reach through the mask! (p. 397)

That is difficult with some players such as Rick – or Richard Cory. They constantly dissemble, namely from themselves. However, like Rick's therapist, we have to "reach through the mask."

Individuals like Rick are people of mystery. Litman's psychological autopsies (1995) of the Richard Cory type of suicide revealed that people often knew little about them. No one knew who Richard Cory was. People only saw the "glitter," "the grace" – or to use Shneidman's term, "the mask." Litman (1995) noted how even wives and partners knew little about them. That was true about Rick's parents, when they were subsequently interviewed. They did not even know about Gloria. Litman described the Richard Cory type as autonomous, independent, self-sufficient, and help rejecting. That was true for Rick although the self-sufficient, independence, and autonomy are false; they are, in fact, people with the opposite characteristic. The self-sufficient and so forth are self-believing masks. The help rejecting, of course, is a hallmark, as Freud (1939/1874e) had documented, of a person with a weak ego, not being able to cope. Inhibition, forgetting, avoidance, and phobia are negative ways to cope to life's demands (Freud, 1939/1974e). Despite Rick being at the therapist's office, he was not in treatment. There was a lack of attachment (Leenaars, 1994). He rejected help, being only there because of a court order. He rejected everything.

Litman (1995) noted that people have a hard time accepting the Richard Cory suicide as a suicide. That was true with Rick. His therapist, the parole officer, and his friends did not accept it, despite the physical evidence. Rick was a mask; he dissembled. But did he kill himself without warning?

A CONCLUDING REMARK

Is it possible to help Rick or Richard Cory? Can we reach through the mask (see Leenaars, Maltsberger, & Neimeyer, 1994)? Shneidman's (1994) guidance here may assist:

> How can the helper reach inside, except through the mask? What this means in practice is that if we have the least reasonable suspicion that a friend or a patient is dormantly suicidal, we have a responsibility to reach behind social and public masks and to touch the real face of suffering. In such a case; the key questions – those that reflect our interest (and paradigmatically, our lifesaving concern) – are "What is going on?" and "Where do you hurt?" The challenge is to resonate to the other's hidden psychache (Shneidman, 1993) to reassemble what the others have dissembled. (p. 397)

Rick's therapist asked "What is wrong?" and "Where do you hurt?" Yet, despite aspiring rescue, Rick felt doomed. There will be, sadly, casualties. There are hazards to doing psychotherapy with suicidal people (Jobes & Maltsberger, 1995).

Only eight out of ten people leave clues about suicide risk. In the other two out of ten, suicide happens without warning. It is generally difficult to predict suicide in people because it is rare. Most suicidal patients do not dissemble; likely less than 20% – maybe as few as 2%. We need, thus, to constantly address the dissembling in this small but lethal group of patients.

REFERENCES

Allport, G. (1942). *The use of personal documents in psychological science.* New York: Social Science Research Council.

American Psychiatric Association. (1994). *Diagnostic and statistical manual of mental disorders* (4th ed.). Washington, DC: Author.

Bongar, B., & Greaney, S. (1994). Essential clinical and legal issues when working with suicidal people. In A. Leenaars, J. Maltsberger, & R. Neimeyer (Eds.), *Treatment of suicidal people* (pp. 179–194). Washington, DC: Taylor & Francis.

Erikson, E. (1963). *Childhood and society* (2nd ed.). New York: W. W. Norton.

Erikson, E. (1980). *Identity and the life cycle.* New York: W. W. Norton.

Exner, J. (1986). *The Rorschach: A comprehensive system*, Vol. 1 (2nd ed.). New York: Wiley.

Fenichel, O. (1954). *The psychoanalytic theory of neurosis.* New York: W. W. Norton.

Frager, R., & Fadiman, J. (1984). *Personality and personal growth* (2nd ed.). New York: Harper & Row.

Friedman, P. (1967). *On suicide.* New York: International Universities Press. (Original work published 1910).

Freud, S. (1974a). General theory of neurosis. In J. Strachey (Ed. & Trans), *The standard edition of the complete psychological works of Sigmund Freud* (Vol. 16, pp. 24–83). London: Hogarth Press. (Original work published 1917)

Freud, S. (1974b). Mourning and melancholia. In J. Strachey (Ed. & Trans), *The standard edition of the complete psychological works of Sigmund Freud* (Vol. 14, pp. 239–260). London: Hogarth Press. (Original work published 1917)

Freud, S. (1974c). A case of homosexuality in a woman. In J. Strachey (Ed. & Trans), *The standard edition of the complete psychological works of Sigmund Freud* (Vol. 18, pp. 147–172). London: Hogarth Press. (Original work published 1920)

Freud, S. (1974d). Group psychology and the analysis of the ego. In J. Strachey (Ed. & Trans.), *The standard edition of the complete psychological works of Sigmund Freud* (Vol. 18, pp. 67–147). London: Hogarth Press. (Original work published 1921)

Freud, S. (1974e). Moses and monotheism. In J. Strachey (Ed. & Trans.), *The standard edition of the complete psychological works of Sigmund Freud* (Vol. 23, pp. 3–137). London: Hogarth Press. (Original work published 1939)

Freud, S. (1974f). An outline of psycho-analysis. In J. Strachey (Ed. & Trans.), *The standard edition of the complete psychological works of S. Freud* (Vol. 23, pp. 137–207). London: Hogarth Press. (Original work published 1940)

Garrison, C., Lewinsohn, P., Marsteller, F., Langhinrichsen, J., & Lann, I. (1991). The assessment of suicidal behavior in adolescents. *Suicide & Life-Threatening Behavior, 21*, 217-230.

Goffman, E. (1974). *Frame analysis*. New York: Harper Colophon.

Goldblatt, M. (1992). *Richard Cory suicides: Diagnostic questions*. Paper presented at the annual conference of the American Association of Suicidology, Chicago, IL.

Hartmann, H. (1939). *Ego psychology and the problem of adaptation*. New York: International Universities Press.

Jobes, D., & Maltsberger, J. (1995). The hazards of treating suicide patients. In M. Sussman (Ed.), *A perilous calling: The hazards of psychotherapy practice* (pp. 200-214). New York: Wiley.

Kimmel, D. (1974). *Adulthood and aging*. New York: Wiley.

Klerman, G. (Ed.) (1986). *Suicide and depression among adolescents and young adults*. Washington, DC: American Psychiatric Press.

Leenaars, A. (1988). *Suicide notes*. New York: Human Sciences Press.

Leenaars, A. (1989). Are young adult's suicides psychologically different from those of other adults? (The Shneidman Lecture). *Suicide & Life-Threatening Behavior, 19*, 249-263.

Leenaars, A. (1991). Suicide in the young adult. In A. Leenaars (Ed.), *Life-span perspectives of suicide* (pp. 121-136). New York: Plenum.

Leenaars, A. (1993). Unconscious processes. In A. Leenaars (Ed.), *Suicidology: Essays in honor of Edwin Shneidman* (pp. 124-147). Northvale, NJ: Aronson.

Leenaars, A. (1994). Crisis intervention with highly lethal suicidal people. In A. Leenaars, J. Maltsberger, & R. Neimeyer (Eds.), *Treatment of suicidal people* (pp. 45-59). Washington, DC: Taylor & Francis.

Leenaars, A. (1996). Suicide: A multidimensional malaise. *Suicide & Life-Threatening Behavior, 26*, 221-236.

Leenaars, A., Balance, W., Pellarin, S., Aversano, G., Magli, A., & Wenckstern, S. (1988). Facts and myths of suicide in Canada. *Death Studies, 12*, 191-210.

Leenaars, A., & Lester, D. (Eds.) (1996). *Suicide & the unconscious*. Northvale, NJ: Aronson.

Leenaars, A., Maltsberger, J., & Neimeyer, R. (Eds.). (1994). *Treatment of suicidal people*. Washington, DC: Taylor & Francis.

Lester, D. (1992). *Why people kill themselves?* (3rd ed.). Springfield IL: Thomas.

Levinson, D. (1986). Development in the novice phase of early development. In G. Klerman (Ed.), *Suicide and depression among adolescents and young adults* (pp. 1-15). Washington, DC: American Psychiatric Press.

Litman, R. (1967). Sigmund Freud on suicide. In E. Shneidman (Ed.), *Essays in self-destruction* (pp. 324-344). New York: Aronson.

Litman, R. (1995). *Suicide without a clue*. Paper presented at the annual conference of the American Association of Suicidology, Phoenix, AZ.

Maltsberger, J. (1986). *Suicide risk: The formulation of clinical judgment*. New York: New York University Press.

McIntosh, J., Hubbard, R., & Santos, J. (1983). *Suicide facts and myths: A compilation and study of prevalence*. Paper presented at the annual conference of the American Association of Suicidology, Dallas, TX.

Meissner, W. (1981). *Internalization in psychoanalysis*. New York: International Universities Press.

Menninger, K. (1938). *Man against himself*. New York: Harcourt, Brace.

Michel, K. (1988). Suicide in young people is different. *Crisis, 9*, 135-145.

Murray, H. (1967). Death to the world: The passions of Herman Melville. In E. Shneidman (Ed.), *Essays in self-destruction* (pp. 7-29). New York: Science House.

Neugarten, B., Moore, J., & Lowe, J. (1965). Age norms, age constraints, and adult socialization. *American Journal of Sociology, 70*, 710-717.

Rickgarn, R. (1994). *Perspectives in college student suicide*. Amityville, NY: Baywood.

Robinson, E. (1953). Richard Cory. In L. Thompson (Ed.), *Tilbury Town: Selected poems of Edwin Arlington Robinson*. New York: MacMillan.

Shneidman, E. (1985). *Definition of suicide*. New York: Wiley.

Shneidman, E. (1993). *Suicide as psychache*. Northvale, NJ: Aronson.

Shneidman, E. (1994). Clues to suicide reconsidered. *Suicide & Life-Threatening Behavior, 24*, 395-397.

Shneidman, E., & Farberow, N. (Eds.). (1957). *Clues to suicide*. New York: McGraw-Hill.

Shneidman, E., & Mandelkorn, P. (1970). How to prevent suicide. In E. Shneidman, N. Farberow, & R. Litman (Eds.), *The psychology of suicide* (pp. 125-143). New York: Science House.

Sullivan, H. (1962). Schizophrenia as a human process. In H. Perry, N. Gorvell, & M. Gibbens (Eds.), *The collected works of Harry Stack Sullivan* (Vol. 2). New York: W. W. Norton.

Sullivan, H. (1964). The fusion of psychiatry and social sciences. In H. Perry, N. Gorvell, & M. Gibbens (Eds.), *The collected works of Harry Stack Sullivan*. New York: W. W. Norton.

Zilboorg, G. (1936). Suicide among civilized and primitive races. *American Journal of Psychiatry, 92*, 1347-1369.

3
Culture and Ego-Ideal in Suicide: An Adult Case

John T. Maltsberger, MD

A case is presented in which the patient's self-expectations, arising from his ego ideal, were violated by a conflict with his wife, who came from a different culture and did not share his marital and family values. When she left him he was devastated, not only by the loss of his family, but by the destruction of his ideal vision of himself as a husband and father. A dangerous suicide attempt followed. The psychodynamic formulation of the case and the treatment that followed from it are discussed.

The importance of conscience in suicide has long been appreciated, but greater attention has been paid to its action in self-hate phenomena than to its role in the failure of self-love. Freud (1917/1966a) pointed out 80 years ago how self-attack in depression proceeds through the superego, and every clinical worker who struggles against patients' press to suicide has been impressed with the deadly force of scornful fury turned against the self.

Conscience, or superego, themes other than self-hate have not been neglected in psychoanalytic writing but they have not received so much attention. One of these themes, the place of the ego-ideal in suicide, is the subject of this discussion.

If the self is to cohere, to maintain its integrity under stress, a certain modicum of positive self-regard must be maintained. When this minimum amount of positive self-regard, or self-love (called narcissism in psychoanalysis) is lost, the psychological experience of giving up on oneself ensues. Without a steady base level of narcissism, a depressed patient withdraws any interest from him/herself, so that a kind of inner abandonment occurs, and the self is left without shelter from the bitter winds of self-scorn. Suicide often follows when a patient feels that life is just not worth fighting for any longer. The importance of self-love for self-survival was noticed by Freud (1923/1966b) and later elaborated by Schafer (1960).

In psychoanalytic theory the mental operations involved in maintaining a positive self-regard are treated as a matter of the relationship between the ego (ego in the sense of the self) and a department of the superego system called the *ego-ideal*. The ego-ideal is that agency of the mind that arises from identification with beloved parents, their substitutes, and collective ideals. It constitutes a model toward which a person reaches and attempts to conform; when comparison of the self with the ego-ideal is reasonably approximated, the person will feel good about him/herself (Laplanche & Pontalis, 1973, pp. 144–145). That is to say, a positive narcissistic balance is maintained because conscience approves, or even loves us, when we can experience ourselves as being reasonably like our ideal selves (Murray, 1964).

This discussion is a part of a symposium intended to show transcultural influences in suicidal phenomena. Of the many places where psychoanalytic light might be shed in today's symposium, ego-ideal development and failure is undoubtedly one. The personal qualities of beloved parents, their substitutes, and collective ideals are all colored by the culture in which a child is raised. Ego-ideal is culturally shaped.

John T. Maltsberger is with the Harvard Medical School, Boston. Address correspondence to 38 Fuller Street, Brookline, MA 02146.

PIETER L.: A CASE OF NEAR SUICIDE

Pieter L. was a 47-year-old academic chemist at the time I first met him. He had been admitted to a psychiatric hospital after overdosing on sleeping medicines and locking himself in a garage where he left his car running, intending to go to sleep and die.

About a month before, returning to his suburban home after a week's absence at a professional meeting, he was shocked to find his wife and children gone, the house emptied of furniture, and a note from his wife pinned to the door. It said, "I am getting a divorce, you will hear from my lawyer." He fell into a panic, searched the neighborhood, called the minister, and telephoned all his wife's friends trying to find his family, but to no avail. He overdosed on some over-the-counter medicines and slept for many hours. After waking up, he became increasingly depressed and despondent over the next few weeks. His wife had cleared out all the bank accounts. Served papers by a lawyer, he learned that his wife had obtained a restraining order against him, claiming to the court he was a danger to her and the children. She concealed her whereabouts. He could not go to work. Had a neighbor not grown suspicious when he heard the sounds of an automobile engine in the closed garage late at night and alerted the police, the patient would certainly have died. Rescued, he was taken to a psychiatric hospital against his wishes.

Past History

The patient was born in Belgium near the Netherlands border toward the close of the Second World War. The eldest child of a farm family, he had a brother two years younger and a sister five years younger. His parents were extremely rigid Protestants who valued hard work, family loyalty, and learning, and believed that woman's place was in the home. The younger brother, Hendrik, was the sickly and overprotected favorite of the mother.

Life on the farm was difficult. It was not a prosperous one, and the patient had to do heavy manual work from the time he was 11. The war had been stressful; Pieter's father had on one occasion been beaten up by German soldiers and narrowly escaped deportation. Emotionally the household was undemonstrative and cold. The mother had no sense of humor and was the dominant parent in the house. Strict and demanding, she tolerated no mischief. Pieter's father was exhausted by the heavy work of the farm and was emotionally rather distant.

Pieter was an unusually intelligent, hardworking student. When he reached adolescence the family was persuaded by the minister to release him from the farm to accept a scholarship to a church school. The school was an extremely repressive one where rigid Protestant values were enforced and misbehavior was punished with caning. It was a good school academically, however, and Pieter excelled, especially in the classics and in science. Graduating from the school at the top of his class, his pleasure was cut short by an abrupt confrontation with his parents.

They told him that as he was the brighter son, he could no longer look to them for support; nor could he live on the farm unless he wanted to be a full-time field laborer. The younger, favored brother, Hendrik, less gifted academically, was to be given the farm as his inheritance, and Pieter was to receive nothing. The parents believed Pieter could look after himself in the future and that the younger brother could not. That this decision was primarily his mother's, Pieter had little doubt. His father said little in this interview but sadly supported his wife. Thus Pieter was deprived of his share of the farm as a reward for his hard work and achievement. But he was also given a vote of confidence about his native strength and capacity for survival that Hendrik was not.

Pieter accepted this bitter news without protest. He obtained a scholarship to the university and, after graduating, was able to come to the United States to a prominent institution on the West Coast for graduate studies in chemistry. Again he excelled. Shortly before obtaining his doctorate he met and fell in love with Clara, a pretty, vivacious woman 15 years younger than he. Her parents were divorced and she had never been able to settle down to steady academic work, but what did it matter? Pieter felt he had degrees enough for them both; he would bring her along intellectually. He adored her; her warmth and beauty, he said retrospectively, seemed to take the chill out of his North European bones. After some initial ambivalence and flattered by his devotion, she decided to accept his worship, married him, and looked forward to raising an ideal family.

Pieter and Clara moved to another part of the United States where he received a faculty appointment at another prestigious university. He worked very hard and rapidly rose toward tenure. He published regularly and rapidly made a name for himself as a promising, creative scientist. But things did not go well at home. Clara had quickly become pregnant, had a child, a boy, and then was pregnant again in only a few months. A second son was born. A year and a half later, there was a third baby, this time a daughter. She felt overwhelmed and restless. Three children in diapers were more than she could manage. She grew depressed and irritable. She blamed Pieter that he was not "more supportive." She resented the lists of books he suggested she should read. She wanted paid household help, time out with her friends, and jazz concerts. She was not sure what she wanted to do with her life; marriage and motherhood were disappointing. Perhaps she would go back for further university studies, she said, or perhaps become a professional photographer. She enrolled in a number of expensive programs but completed none of them. In the midst of this domestic turmoil Pieter's father died of cancer of the colon; Pieter suspected the family doctor had given him a lethal injection so as not to prolong his illness.

Pieter could not understand his wife. His unspoken assumption had been that she would stay home, raise the children, cook the meals, encourage him, and keep quiet—just as he had understood family living in Belgium. Clara next began to be interested in the women's liberation movement.

Pieter, Clara, and the children had always attended church. Then, to his horror, their church added a young woman assistant to the staff who promptly organized a woman's "study group" that took up such matters as battered women, women's oppression, and the proper place of women in the family and the workplace.

Pieter was angry that his meals were rarely ready on time, that the housekeeping was careless, and that Clara was increasingly critical of him. Their sexual relationship deteriorated. One day he told Clara she was just like Madame Bovary in Flaubert's novel.

Conflict in the house increased, and though he usually controlled his temper, he often looked grim and ready to explode. She decided he would soon begin to beat her. Clara misinterpreted his roughhousing with the boys as abusive. When he grabbed her playfully one day she screamed and ran out of the house, calling out to the neighbors to help her. Though he had a good relationship with the children, Pieter was a strict father. He insisted on a heavy schedule of chores, rigorous attention to homework, and academic application. Academic performance did not seem so important to Clara; she advocated greater freedom for children. Influenced by their mother's fears of Pieter's anger, they began to withdraw from and avoid their father. All three became rebellious about homework.

In this context Pieter left town for his professional meeting, only to return home to find himself abandoned and alone.

Treatment

When first admitted to the hospital the patient was somewhat but not profoundly depressed; he was certainly hostile and bitterly suicidal. Pieter very much looked the academic; dressed in flannels and tweeds, he was a tall, well-developed man with horn-rimmed glasses. On the ward he kept himself busy making notes on his laptop computer and reading professional journals. He said his wife's behavior was totally beyond his comprehension but slowly over several weeks accepted the fact she would not return to him. His life was over, he said, and having nothing to live for, he would certainly kill himself as soon as he was discharged, no matter how long he was kept in the hospital.

Efforts to see the wife and to establish a visiting schedule with the children were fruitless. She agreed to one interview only, when she proved determined to go forward with the divorce and quite paranoid in her attitude toward her husband. She was near delusional in her belief he would attack her or the children, though he had never done so. Through legal maneuvers she blocked the children's visiting their father. Pieter became quite embittered against his children; though they were young, he said he expected better of them. They were no better than traitors to their father and had been corrupted by their mother with her American values and contempt for the ties and obligations of marriage and family, he said. In his rigid way, he refused to fight in the courts for visiting rights.

The patient agreed to accept antidepressant medicines but was hostile and devaluative toward most of the psychiatrists. He was, nevertheless, able to develop a kind of bantering camaraderie with me, partly because I would repay his "black" humor in kind and challenged his efforts to devaluate me. He began to respond to the antidepressant medicines and one day he said, towering over me, "You're not such a bad little old guy, but this is an ignorant racket you are in, and why don't you admit you're just a drug pusher?" He was shocked, embarrassed, and not a little pleased when I retorted, "Is that the way you treat your friends? Ignorant? Well, I'm not through with you yet, and as far as those pills are concerned, you had better take them and be grateful. With the help of the pills I intend to drag you up out of this mess. When are you going to wake up, quit this suicide talk, and take the loss of your family like a man instead of a whimpering coward?"

Strong talk, you may say. Spoken angrily, or at the wrong time, without a positive relationship with the patient, such talk could be destructive. But this intervention was based on a diagnosis of the patient's ego-ideal difficulties and marked the beginning of an effective therapeutic alliance. He knew I cared about him and that I was firmly on the side of his living. That he had pitched himself into a state of self-pity and lost his adult perspective was a stinging new idea that took hold.

The patient certainly had exhibited the familiar turning of anger against himself. He blamed himself for being a fool in marrying Clara in the first place, but he still loved her and he experienced little subjective anger against her. He was giving himself an emotional caning. The anger-against-self problem softened under the influence of antidepressant medicines to a considerable degree, but the patient had effectively given up on living, and this the medicines did not touch. He demanded of life and of himself certain conditions without which he was not prepared to carry on – he insisted on a family very much of the same kind in which he had grown up. The loss of his wife and children in such a brutally shocking way had destroyed any sense of pride or achievement he had. His success as a scientist was not enough to sustain him. Quite apart from what he felt for his lost wife and children, the patient lost a part of himself in their departure – he lost himself as a powerful, effective *pater familias*; this sense of himself was essential to his narcissistic balance, and he could not go on without it.

In ego-ideal terms, the formula might read like this: "Thou shalt marry, father a family, and establish a stable bourgeois life in which hard work, loyalty, and academic performance are valued and pursued by all. Fail in this, and you are not a man. If you fail, the responsibility of the failure will be all yours, because a real man knows how to keep his wife and children in order." Living in an empty house and shut off from Clara and the children, the patient was riven from his self-ideal, and he had given up on himself. Lacking much capacity to love himself (he had not been much loved as a child), he was desolated by the loss of Clara, who had helped dispel "the chill in his bones." Convinced his life was not worth saving, he was angry and rejecting toward any professional staff who attempted to interfere.

I saw the therapeutic task as one of ego-ideal modification, necessary if the patient were to survive. I recognized the following tasks:

1. Restoration of capacity for at least minimal positive self-regard. This would require changing some self-expectations.
2. Strengthening the patient's capacity to endure the painful feelings of loss without surrendering to despair.
3. Relinquishing the omnipotent self-belief that the breakdown of his marriage proved he was not a man.
4. Softening his rigid view that if he did not create a perfect European bourgeois family in America, whatever the obstacles, he was worthless.

A major obstacle was the patient's tendency to devaluate anybody who tried to interfere with his hopeless life view. Because I was prepared actively to challenge his hopelessness and despair, the patient was annoyed, but he was also very surprised. He was deeply moved to discover that I genuinely cared about him and could not be frightened off by his contempt or sarcasm. My "tough" stance was somewhat like that of a marine sergeant or a football coach who was determined to pull a rookie through–loving but demanding, not standing for guff. In effect, I offered myself as an auxiliary external ego-ideal and invited the patient's respect and idealization by showing him I knew something about living that he did not. I became available as an exterior resource that he might use, through identification, to establish a less rigid and more forgiving ego-ideal.

My suggestion that suicide as a solution was a coward's way out immediately appealed to the patient's powerful capacity to stand up to adversity *if he had a mind to do it*, as he had done in his youth. I pointed out to him that when Hitler's forces overran France, the Netherlands, and Belgium, and gave his father a beating, his father stood up to the hard times and did not "run off and commit suicide." The battle was thereby immediately enjoined over whether suicide was self-respecting or not.

He insisted that my attitude toward suicide–that it hardly ever makes mature sense–was just professional dogmatism. He challenged me, claiming I knew little about suffering. By this time discharged from the hospital, he made a visit to his family in Belgium and returned in two weeks, triumphantly telling me that he had discussed his possible suicide with his mother and his brother Hendrik, and that both of them had given their permission for him to do it if he felt that was best. He said people in the Low Countries had a different attitude to suicide than Americans, and that he was not going to let me Americanize him. Had not his own father died of a lethal injection when he no longer wanted to suffer?

The patient was delighted when I would have none of his so-called "European" ideas about suicide. I told him that he was not terminally ill, that he was just "raising hell" because life had given him a hard knock, and that I greatly admired the strength and courage of *real* European manhood, to which he was called, but from which he was shrinking. Since when had his mother and Hendrik really cared that much about him, anyway, I asked him. He began to settle into psychotherapy.

The patient began to weep when I showed him the parallels between his rejection by Clara and his parents' (mother's) disinheriting him. He drew comfort from memories of his courageous father who had suffered through the war and grieved his death for the first time. He was impressed with stories I told him of others' lives, of men who had suffered through equivalent losses, or worse, who had survived and gone on to rebuild their lives. His sorrow over the loss of the idealized Clara was especially poignant as he remembered how lovely she had been in the early years of their marriage, before she turned against him. He hated to cry in my presence but became increasingly able to do so as I supported and teased him into a new attitude: that only the brave can truly grieve. Had not the great Achilles, I reminded him, wept over the loss of a friend?

He began to grow angry at Clara. Though he never came to understand how she could have behaved so incomprehensibly, he stopped blaming himself that he had not been able to build a Belgian family in the contemporary culture of the United States where everything is changing and traditional roles for men and women are fluid. He began to see how he and Clara had married when she was still very immature, and that she had never shared the European family values he had taken for granted and so much cherished.

He began to take a new interest in his work, and slowly his depression lifted. We worked together twice a week for about two years, and it took about 18 months for the patient to emerge from true suicide danger. Competitive and scrappy to the last, the patient insisted to the end of our treatment that he reserved the right to commit suicide one day if that seemed the best thing for him to do. But the sting had gone out of the threat, and at the time we parted company, he had a twinkle in his eye and spring in his step. He has left the city where his family was so tragically disrupted and moved abroad, where he has obtained another academic appointment. Though fearful, he is hopeful and feeling a renewed interest in women. "But not in American women," he declares.

CONCLUSION

This patient, with a harsh superego demanding extremely high, even impossible personal and professional achievement, and with little inner capacity to maintain an attitude of positive self-regard (he had not been much loved as a child), expected of himself that—against the forces of the prevailing culture of the United States and in spite of the ambivalence of his wife—he should be able to establish a bourgeois family along rigid Belgian Protestant lines and to raise his children accordingly. When his marriage collapsed a suicide attempt followed.

The patient's recovery depended on an active, engaging psychotherapeutic style in which the patient's devaluative transference attitudes were challenged, idealization of the therapist invited, and positive emotional support provided. The heart of the work lay in helping the patient recognize that his self-expectations respecting a family were impossible, at least in his present cultural circumstances. He was able to grieve the loss of his wife and children, and to leave the United States, wary but hopeful for the future.

REFERENCES

Freud, S. (1966a). Mourning and melancholia. In J. Strachey (Ed. and Trans.), *The standard edition of the complete psychological works of Sigmund Freud* (Vol. 14, pp. 239–258). London: Hogarth Press. (Original work published 1917)

Freud, S. (1966b). The ego and the id. In J. Strachey (Ed. and Trans.), *The standard edition of the complete psychological works of Sigmund Freud* (Vol. 19, pp. 3–66). London: Hogarth Press. (Original work published 1923)

Laplanche, J., & Pontalis, J.-B. (1973). *The language of psychoanalysis* (D. Nicholson-Smith, Trans.). New York: W. W. Norton.

Murray, J. M. (1964). Narcissism and the ego ideal. *Journal of the American Psychoanalytic Association, 12*, 477–511.

Schafer, R. (1960). The loving and beloved superego in Freud's structural theory. *Psychoanalytic Study of the Child, 15*, 163–188.

4
Being Suicidal and Elderly in Changing Times: A Case History

Joseph Richman, PhD

Mr. Andrew A, at age 67, is a physically well and mentally active man who is involved in business failures and marital conflicts, which brought him dangerously close to precipitating his own demise. He is different from my other elderly suicidal patients, most of whom were ill, disabled, and in decline. They were grieving for many reasons, such as the loss of a spouse or – frequently – themselves as they had been. Andrew's story has hopeful implications for the changing nature of aging and suicide that extend beyond himself as an individual or my interventions as a therapist.

CASE HISTORY

I received a call from a physician, asking if I could see a patient who told the doctor that he wanted to commit suicide. Suicidal people in my experience are the best and most rewarding psychotherapy patients, and I was happy to oblige. Andrew, the patient, phoned within an hour, and we made an appointment to see him and his wife the next day. He was an American-born man of Jewish origin, who was eager to talk and welcomed the opportunity to meet with me. I saw him in a combination of individual and marital therapy for two months, and for individual therapy which has been ongoing for the past two years.

Andrew was an informally dressed, gray-haired man who appeared his stated age. His first words, "I should have done this 30 years ago," foretold a developmental crisis around aging. He was a businessman and a professional, currently unemployed, with a history of failed business ventures. He said that he was having a complete nervous breakdown. "I can't work. I can't sleep. I keep thinking of suicide. It's because of my wife. We had a little disagreement; she's a very nervous woman and makes a big deal out of nothing. She said she is going to get a divorce and ordered me to leave the house."

His wife was an attractive, youthful-looking woman, an executive in a large firm. Her first husband had died suddenly five years ago. She became depressed and agitated, with suicidal impulses that made her afraid to go into the kitchen near a knife. Andrew was a friend of her husband's. After his death, Andrew was solicitous and in tune with her feelings and needs. He remained that way throughout most of their marriage and has been a great comfort to her. She declared that she could not have survived without him.

Mrs. A was the breadwinner from the beginning of their marriage. She bought the home they are living in. She put a $60,000 bank account in both their names. A few days ago, she went to the bank to withdraw some money and was told that the account was closed. The money had been gradually withdrawn by her husband. When she confronted Andrew with the situation, he explained that he had been arranging a business deal, but that it failed.

There had been problems and many quarrels around money throughout their marriage, but now, she said, she had had it. She began to realize how secretive he

Joseph Richman is Professor Emeritus, Albert Einstein College of Medicine; and in private practice, New York. Address correspondence to the author at 50 Earley Street, Bronx, NY 10464.

Suicide and Life-Threatening Behavior, Vol. 27(1), Spring 1997

was about his life and career, and that he had never discussed his business dealings with her.

Mr. A promised to be more open and to respect her money. She should realize, he added, that he loves her. She replied that she loves him too and is terrified at the prospect of being alone without him. She agreed to reconsider the divorce and hoped that therapy would help him turn over a new leaf.

This was Mr. A's fourth marriage. The previous marriages had been marked by constant quarrels over money and failed business deals. According to his daughter, Mr. A's father had been a distant and depressed man, while Mr. A's mother had been an eccentric woman, a New Age mystic many years before it was fashionable, and a Christian Scientist. The parents had different and largely incompatible personalities.

ASSESSMENT

Suicidal thoughts and impulses were a prominent part of Andrew's presenting complaints. During the arguments with his wife, he often had the urge to throw himself out the window at the height of the quarrel. He was thinking of getting back at his wife by leaving his insurance to her. Some readers may find it incomprehensible that a man would kill himself and by so doing benefit his wife, as a form of revenge. That is part of the logic of suicide, as Shneidman and Farberow (1970) pointed out. Mr. A talked as though he would be present to see how sorry and guilty his wife would feel as a result of his suicide.

My initial diagnostic impression was of a bipolar disorder. However, his speech was intellectualized rather than pressured. The failures in his career and his irresponsible behavior with his wife's money and property had a repetitive, compulsive quality. He revealed a preoccupation with death, combined with a strong although denied pessimistic attitude. His affect and ideation suggested an underlying chronic depression, related to unresolved mourning.

His negative thinking was chronic but related now to feelings that it was too late and that he was too old. Social supports were limited. He was alienated from his daughter and his wife, and he had no friends of his own. The diagnostic impression, in summary, was of a major depression in an obsessive-compulsive disorder, with decompensating defenses and a moderate to severe risk of suicide.

He had never grieved appropriately for either his mother or his father. Although he was strongly identified with his mother, with a symbiotic tie that continued after her death, his attachment was combined with much ambivalence. My notes to the first session included the statement "The patient exhibits many unresolved problems with his mother, which have probably been repeated with his wives."

While his current disturbed state was precipitated when his wife decided on a divorce and told him to leave, his provocative actions suggested an unconscious need to precipitate the crisis. His lifelong history of maladaptive behavior seemed motivated to preserve and repeat the earlier attachments.

The treatment plan was for outpatient crisis intervention, with the goals of reducing the threat of separation, and arranging for him to work and pay back his debt to his wife.

THERAPY

Throughout treatment, his relationship to me was an ambivalent combination of disengagement and a clinging dependency. He said little about his present circumstances and less about the past, and spent the bulk of the time telling me how good the future will be when his plans work out. Current events were most often revealed through enraged phone calls from his wife, informing me that he had helped himself to money put aside in the house for everyday expenses and similar events, and ending with the words "He'll never change." He met these exposures with a lack of awareness of his own involvement and feelings, almost resembling a hysterical belle indifference, combined with a justification of helping himself to her property.

"She has a lot of money," he said.

"It's her money," I replied. He agreed but added, "She is very nervous."

"She is entitled to be nervous," I said.

"But she faints and falls on the floor," he said.

"She has a right to faint. Why does it bother you so much?"

"I do so much for her."

"You are a very giving person," I agreed. "You just have to be less taking."

He continued to meet his wife's outrage in a relatively bland manner until she again threatened divorce and ordered him out of the house, which precipitated another crisis. He pictured himself as homeless and living in a shelter, and vowed revenge. Suicidal ideation became more prominent; he phoned me frequently at all hours, in an agitated state. He asked for extra sessions, during which he ventilated homicidal as well as suicidal impulses. However, the crisis gradually abated.

The most striking feature during treatment was the symbiotic nature of Andrew's attachments. Symbiotic relationships originate in a symbiotic family system (Richman, 1986), where two people see themselves as merged rather than as separate entities. At the same time, at least one other family member is detached and seemingly disengaged. That member plays an intrinsic role in the symbiotic system, and psychotherapy reveals that the disengaged other partner is anything but detached. The major function of symbiotic relationships is to avoid the painful process of grieving by symbolically keeping the earlier symbiotic partner alive. The fear of losing a symbiotic relationship is what makes separation so devastating and destructive in suicidal people.

Andrew repeatedly recalled the special relationship he had with his mother. When he was nine years old she emphasized to him how superior he was to his father. The most frequent phrase he recalled was her statement "Don't tell Daddy." It did not matter what he should not tell, but it preserved the relationship and reversal of generation roles.

Symbiosis can be modified in therapy and its destructive effects diminished, but it must first be accepted. What follows is an example.

One day he walked into my office in an unusually jovial mood. "Hello, Joseph," he said. "Hello, Andrew," I replied, and added, "You know the story of two men in an insane asylum, both of whom believed they were Napoleon. One of them became depressed. The other said, "If I were you, and I am. . . . "

Andrew responded, "I love it!"

Through humor I was recognizing that the family symbiotic pattern had been transferred to me. We were merged. It then became possible to modify the symbiosis in therapy, as something that could be positive as well as destructive. I may note that the positive effects were possible because Andrew possessed the saving grace of a sense of humor. He became more relaxed and gradually more open about his present situation and past experiences.

He started another business, which became successful, as had been true when he began businesses in the past. With a reversal of fortunes that seemed more than coincidental, his wife lost her job, and he became the one supporting her. After the loss of her job, he soothed her fears, as his mother had done, by having her pray with him in a New Age, spiritual manner.

At one of our last sessions he reported that he now has a superb relationship with his wife and that his business is flourishing, but he feels very insecure. That was a change because he was expressing his own feelings, rather than through his wife. His anxiety was also expressed directly for the first time. He said that he is afraid he will mess up his career again.

He returned to the theme of regrets that he did not go into treatment 30 years ago. He recalled how he would build up one business after another and, just as he was about to close a big deal, do something to offend his clients, whereupon the business would go under. His father had a similar pattern of building up a business and failing. I asked if he thought his father had a problem with Andrew being successful. He replied that he thought so. I then asked if he had a problem in being more successful than his father. He replied that it could be.

I think I moved too fast and pushed too soon for insight. Andrew became fearful of losing the family pattern he had been trying to keep alive, especially the treasured but secret relationship with his mother. He suddenly changed his body position, which had been an open one combined with direct eye contact. He folded his arms across his chest, stopped looking at me, and suggested cutting down on our sessions.

Since then he has canceled sessions for various reasons. He declares that he has been too busy running around because of his business to keep his appointments. That is a danger sign. He phones regularly, telling me that his relationship with his wife continues to be excellent, and that money from his business is starting to roll in. Although he states that he wants to resume treatment, I feel uneasy, because that is the behavior that has been described by his wife and his children preceding his self-defeating behavior in the past.

DISCUSSION

The therapist or counselor must possess a point of view with which to approach the patient. It need not be my view, but there must be *a* view. My approach is an eclectic and comprehensive one, in which biological, psychological, social, and family factors are equally considered, depending upon what is required by the nature of the case. However, I emphasize the relationship, which can be considered a case of first among equals (see Richman, 1986, 1993). I emphasize the positive, but as the story of Andrew A illustrated, I am also reality oriented and do not ignore the negative. I deal with whatever the patient is struggling with. In Andrew's case, it was suicidal impulses and a history of self-destructive behavior of at least 35 years' duration. During that time, he destroyed success at work and relationships in marriage and the family.

Confronted with what seemed the impossibility of changing his behavior because of his age, and another breakup of a marriage that contained many positive features, he fell into a state of despair in which there seemed no way out but suicide. He responded positively to therapy yet continued his self-destructive pattern for at least a year. He eventually improved and has continued to do so. He has been doing well in his marriage and his career for over a year.

My contribution to his improvement is based in large part upon my expectation of negative therapeutic reactions to success in treatment, because that is what happens with severely suicidal patients of all ages. I maintained my positive expectations and worked with Andrew through the setbacks as well as the progress.

The interventions by other therapists may differ, and my interventions with other patients may differ, depending upon the individual and the experiential and situational factors of each patient. The therapist must be flexible. Consultation and supervision are necessary when treating suicidal patients, no matter how experienced the therapist.

I still meet regularly with other experienced therapists who have suicidal patients in their practice, in a self-help and peer supervision group.

The precipitants of a suicidal state in the elderly include retirement, illness, reduced income, and losses of roles, relationships, and loved ones. Andrew A was different in many respects, being involved with recent marital conflicts and ongoing business deals. These situations are more frequently found in younger males.

I hypothesize that Andrew as an individual represents a trend in the elderly for the future. Rachel Pruchno remarked that "the life experiences of people reaching old age during the 21st century will be substantially different from those of people who grew old in earlier decades" (Pruchno, 1996, p. 140). The implication for the 21st century is that people will "age" later and "young" longer.

There are implications for developmental theory. Any study of elderly suicide must consider the meaning of the last stage of life, and for that, a life span approach is essential. The precipitants and motives of suicidal patterns are age related (Richman, 1975). They closely resemble the developmental tasks and crises described by Erikson (1950), even though he was not writing about suicide.

According to Erikson (1950) a perception of failure in old age leads to stagnation, a state of disgust, despair, and grief for a life unfulfilled. That is basically what Antoon Leenaars (1988, 1992) found in his investigations. He studied the suicide notes of young, middle-aged, and older adults from a psychodynamic and developmental perspective. Through his analysis, Leenaars vividly described the existential state of the suicidal elderly just before they killed themselves. In the older suicides, he found a state of despair and a loss of integrity, where "all was a waste" and all was meaningless.

Success and positive resolution, on the other hand, lead to generativity, ego integrity, and wisdom. The elder can review his or her entire life, see it as a unified gestalt, and find it good. With integrity there is serenity and readiness, a sense of consolation and completeness. Our total existence is a work of art like a painting or a symphony. Suicide, however, leaves this great work forever unfinished.

Leenaars did not find integrity, success, or wisdom, but only hopelessness in the suicide notes of the older adults. In his only word on the subject of suicide, Erikson (Jacobs, Brown, & Erikson, 1989) could offer only a few scattered speculations. It was Leenaars' findings that validated Erik Erikson's concepts, as applied to the suicidal elderly.

Suicide is the result of despair, never of self-affirmation. Fortunately, the life span concepts of Leenaars and Erikson are of inestimable value in understanding how the elderly can be worked with in psychotherapy, to the very end of life.

Development occurs in a family and social context. Ego integrity is not a solitary process, nor is despair, the dark, self-destructive component of old age. They involve others. The social and interpersonal aspects are behind the effectiveness of psychotherapy for the elderly, for the suicidal, and even for the terminally ill. Dedicated psychotherapists have not only treated the terminally ill but have reduced pain and terror, resolved family conflicts, and helped the patients to achieve a state of peace and acceptance at the end of life (Richman, 1995).

The implication for psychotherapy is the need to recognize the potential for growth and development of the elderly and apply this recognition to their treatment. We still have a lot to learn in order to find and apply the optimal treatment methods that go beyond palliative care. The growth and development of therapy requires a working alliance of research and clinical professionals, to keep pace with the growth and developmental potentials of the despairing and suicidal elderly.

Freud said that the hallmark of maturity is the ability to love and to work. Andrew A's story suggests that the tasks of work and love will continue, and even overlap with the last stages of life, the periods associated with generativity and ego integrity. Men and women will continue to be involved in active and developing intimate relationships and career activities.

Margot Tallmer and I observed a similar trend during a (as yet unpublished) study of humor. Dr. Tallmer collected jokes from elderly people in New York, and we analyzed the material as an expression of the interests, attitudes, and life tasks of the elderly. We found that marital, sexual, and work problems were frequent themes, up to age 75. Those are the same themes that are given by younger subjects. The humor changed for those over 80, dealing more with sensory decline, memory loss, illness, and death. The stories of many older subjects also revealed a good-humored acceptance of their decline. Since dysfunction was not the center of their attention, they were able to remain active.

I recall Dr. Ida Davidoff, a colleague and sometime coauthor (see Richman & Davidoff, 1971), who is well into her 80s. She described the stages of development as "infancy, childhood, adolescence, youth, middle age, and 'You're looking good.'" Her comment to the cult of youth that pervades our society was , "The reason young people look so good is you couldn't stand them otherwise."

The results of our humor study are consistent with Andrew A, active and involved in a relatively new business, and with many changes taking place in his life. Andrew's story is also consistent with the optimistic prediction that middle age in the next millennium will last longer, while old age will also last longer but start later. Health, energy, and an engagement in life and relationships will be among the gifts of an increase in the life span.

There have been many predictions about elderly suicide in the 21st century, many of them dire. They point out the expected increase in the elderly population, the group with the highest suicide rate. There is evidence of a higher rate of depression in the baby boomers born after World War II, who are the elderly of the next millennium. And we all know that untreated or unimproved depression is associated with suicide.

The news media have attributed the rising elderly suicide rate in the 1980s to the biomedical advances that allowed people to live longer but to be miserable while doing so. It should be noted, however, that these biomedical gains began well before 1980, and that they enable people to be healthy and active longer. While the number of elderly has increased dramatically, as Abeles, Gift, and Ory (1994) pointed out, the amount of illness and disability is actually less than had been predicted. I attribute the lack of attention to the positive results of biomedical advances to an automatic adherence to negative thinking. It is a social lag and clinging to what Paul Krugman (1990) called our "age of diminished expectations."

It is likely that social forces – such as the availability of medical care for all, the fate of agism, and the growth of approval or disapproval of euthanasia for the elderly – will make a greater difference than biomedical progress in the future suicide rate. I am not underestimating the importance of biology and medicine. On the contrary, if social changes combine fruitfully with biomedical advances rather than clashing with them, and if both are dedicated to advancing the well-being of people, the future may be bright for the elderly and everyone.

Whatever changes occur in society, therapy, and people, suicide will not go away. While we cannot directly influence the suicide rate by treating suicidal people and their families, that will not stop us from continuing to treat them successfully. With the expected increase in the elderly populations, there will be a growing need for clinicians to help the suicidal elderly. More educational programs and work with the media are needed to notify the public and professionals about the knowledge, abilities, humor, and other assets of the elderly. The principles involved in reaching an old age of wisdom and ego integrity can be applied to the task of reducing the hopelessness and despair that leads to suicide.

Andrew A may be a forerunner of many more well-functioning elderly. The old-old are the fastest growing population group in our country. However, even the suicidal old-old can be helped to a life that is affirmed and enriched to the very end. Our work can prevent many suicides and in the process even lead to a greater ego integrity in the therapist. Meanwhile, I shall continue to see Andrew.

REFERENCES

Abeles, R. P., Gift, H. C., & Ory, M. G. (Eds.). (1994). *Aging and the quality of life.* New York: Springer.

Erikson, E. H. (1950). *Childhood and society.* New York: Norton.

Jacobs, D., Brown H. N., & Erikson, E. (1989). Foreword: A dialogue with Erik H. Erikson. In D. Jacobs & H. N. Brown (Eds.), *Suicide: Understanding and responding.* Madison, CT: International Universities Press.

Krugman, P. (1990). *The age of diminished expectations.* Cambridge, MA: MIT Press.

Leenaars, A. (1988). *Suicide notes.* New York: Human Sciences Press.

Leenaars, A. (1992). Suicide notes of the older adult. In Leenaars, A. A., Maris R. W., McIntosh, J. L., & Richman, J. (Eds.), *Suicide and the older adult* (pp. 62–79). New York: Guilford Press.

McIntosh, J. L., Santos, J. F., Hubbard, R. W., & Overholser, J. C. (1994). *Elder suicide: Research, theory, and treatment.* Washington, DC: American Psychological Association.

Pruchno, R. A. (1996). Charting new horizons: Living better with age. *Contemporary Psychology, 41,* 138–140.

Richman, J. (1975). *Precipitants and motives of attempted suicide in younger and older subjects.* Paper presented at the Fifth Annual Conference of the International Gerontological Association, Jerusalem, Israel.

Richman, J. (1986). *Family therapy for suicidal people.* New York: Springer.

Richman, J. (1993). *Preventing elderly suicide: Overcoming personal despair, professional neglect, and social bias.* New York: Springer.

Richman, J. (1995). From despair to integrity: An Ericksonian approach to psychotherapy for the terminally ill. *Psychotherapy, 32*(2), 317–322.

Richman, J., & Davidoff, I. (1971). Interaction testing and counseling as a form of crisis intervention during marital therapy. In *Proceedings, 79th Annual Convention, American Psychological Association,* Vol. 6, pp. 439–440.

Shneidman, E. S., & Farberow, N. L. (1970). The logic of suicide. In Shneidman, E. S., Farberow, N. L., & Litman, R. E. (Eds.), *The psychology of suicide.* New York: Science House.

5
Social Suicide

Ronald W. Maris, PhD

At first blush suicide seems like the ultimate private action. However, it is argued that social forces and social pathologies figure prominently in the dynamics of suicide interacting with more individual characteristics. Several examples of "social suicide" (intentional cotemporaneous self-murder of two or more persons) are considered, including mass suicide, organizational self-destruction, social analogues to individual suicide, and military suicide. Suicide prevention requires social, economic, and cultural transformations at the primary prevention level, not just individual psychotherapy and dispensing of the latest antidepressants.

Given the usual focus in suicidology on individuals (especially on private self-destructive intent), what follows may be seen as iconoclastic, even heretical. However, one should always keep an open mind. Could it be that there really are no individual suicides? For example, are the perspectives of adolescents, the elderly, Africans, Chinese, Latin Americans, Canadians, Germans, Japanese, and so on distinctive because of their incremental *social* attributes, not their individual traits?

CONCEPTS AND DEFINITIONS

But we get ahead of ourselves. What is to be understood by the phrase "social suicide" (for a brief history of the sociology of suicide, see Maris, 1989 or 1992). Strictly speaking, any roughly cotemporaneous intentional self-murder of two or more persons qualifies as "social suicide"; examples are the suicide pact of a husband and wife (like Henry Van Dusen and his wife Elizabeth, president of Union Theological Seminary in New York City), the cluster suicides of adolescents (Berman & Jobes, 1991, p. 102 ff.), and most obviously mass suicides, like the 908 to 914 who died in Jonestown, Guyana, in 1978 (Maris, 1996).

Among the candidates for "social suicides" we may need to examine are:

- Mass suicides
- Organizational self-destruction
- Suicide clusters
- Social analogues to individual suicide
- Military suicides and war
- Murder–suicides
- Suicide pacts
- Witnessed suicides

More on some of these examples later on.

What does it mean to be "social"? Dictionary definitions do not help much. For example, the *American Heritage College Dictionary* (1993) says "social" is related to communal living or to society. "Social" is often contrasted with "individual." If so, a social suicide would not be an individual suicide. However, it is hard to think of any purely individual suicides—after all, all human beings have parents, a language, a cultural heritage, at least a rudimentary family, and so on. There really is not a ferral Romulous or Remus suicidal wolf-child.

It is tempting to conclude that suicidal intentions are private, subjective, and radically individual. But are they? Here one is reminded of Austrian linguistic philosopher Ludwig Wittgenstein and his "private language argument" (1953, especially p. 88 ff.). Wittgenstein speculated that since only individuals feel their own pain (or pleasure), perhaps the very meaning of a sensation ("Empfindung") word is

Ronald W. Maris is with the University of South Carolina.

Suicide and Life-Threatening Behavior, Vol. 27(1), Spring 1997

private (1953, p. 92 ff.). After all, only we experience what our personal pain denotes. Consider how we come to use the word "toothache." How does our mother know what exactly we are feeling, when she suggests to us that we have a "toothache"? However, Wittgenstein concluded that the meaning of a word is *not* private, but common and social–it is how the word is used in a language.

Perhaps a schizophrenic suicide resulting from pure dopamine excess or dysfunction would be considered asocial, that is, "just" biological–but even schizophrenic suicides have some distinctive group characteristics. Of course, one could be an idiographic reductionist and argue that every human being is unique and, thus, that every suicide is unique–no other one is quite like it. However, almost no one believes that one suicide is totally unlike all other suicides. If it were, then the science of suicidology would give way to magic or its psychological parallel, clinical judgment.

Usually the concept of the Social involves numbers greater than one (such as Simmel's dyads and triads; see Wolff, 1950, p. 124) and some interaction or exchange among the individuals or units involved. An important characteristic of social interaction is that it changes or transforms individuals. Sociologist Lester Ward (Martindale, 1981, p. 70), coined the concept of *synergy*, or the joint working together of individual components. Often as we move from isolated individuals to collective outcomes, the result is paradoxical. For example, all beneficient individual inputs may result in collective pathology. As German philosopher Goethe wrote (cf. Maris, 1971):

> "Jene Kraft die stets das gute will und stets das Bose schafft"
>
> [that force which constantly wants Good and constantly creates Bad]

The celebrated French social philosopher, Emile Durkheim, wrote most perceptively both about the Social and suicide (1895/1938, 1897/1951). Durkheim believed that social facts, like suicide rates, were not reducible to individuals. He argued that social facts were external to and constraining of individuals. When individuals associated or interacted, the product of their exchanges was qualitatively different from the individuals themselves. In much the same way that water is not the same as two parts hydrogen and one part oxygen, society or suicide is not reducible to the individuals that comprise it. Like Jung's archetypes, Durkheim claimed that the collective conscience was not just the sum of individual consciences. The Social always has an emergent or even transcendent property to it, such that the social sum is not equivalent to the totality of its individual parts. For example, a swiss Rolex watch is not the same as a heap of all of its parts. Those parts have to be integrated in a special way that transforms them into a Rolex. Thus, Durkheim thought that suicide can never be explained by an individual case.

Since suicide rates are generic social regularities, they can only be explained by antecedent social variations. As is well known, Durkheim argued that suicide rates varied inversely with social integration; the more the social integration, the lower the suicide rates. For example, "anomic" suicide occurred when social regularities or norms were abruptly altered, as in the U.S. stock market crash of 1929 or the fairly short time periods in the 20th century in which the U.S. divorce rates rose rapidly. In addition to normative disruption, suicide rates are also exacerbated by excessive isolation or individuation, a condition Durkheim called "egoistic" suicide. In both of the above types of suicide the protective forces of the social are attentuated. Individual traits, Durkheim believed, could not possibly explain suicide rates. Perhaps one reasonable way to proceed now would be to examine individual and social forces in a concrete, historical example of mass suicide.

MASS SUICIDE

So-called mass suicides are an obvious example of social suicides. One of the first mass suicides occurred at Masada (Israel) in 72–73 A.D., when 960 Jewish men, women, and children killed themselves to avoid capture by the Romans (John Mann, a Jewish scholar and noted suicidologist, says the Talmud also records the mass suicides of approximately 200 young men and 200 young women). It was common in the Jewish scriptures to suicide to avoid capture or defeat in battle. Perhaps the best-known mass suicide took place November 18, 1978, when between 908 and 914 followers of evangelist Jim Jones drank cyanide- and depressant-laced Kool-Aid (although a few of the cult were shot to death–including Jones himself) in the jungle of Guyana, South America, at "Jonestown." On April 19, 1993, we also witnessed the deaths of about 85 members of David Koresh's Branch Davidian cult in Waco, Texas (*Fort Worth Star Telegram*, May 12, 1993). These deaths were a mixture of suicides, homicides, and accidents. Most of the cult burned to death, but up to 22 were shot (including Koresh) either by themselves or by federal agents (Federal Bureau of Investigation and Bureau of Alcohol, Tobacco, and Firearms). On October 6, 1994, the Associated Press reported the suffocation, gunshot, and burning suicides of 48 to 53 members of the Order of the Solar Temple cult in Switzerland, and 16 more immolation suicides by solar cult members in France on December 24, 1995.

Among the common characteristics of all of the above mass suicides are the following. First, all of these groups were religious cults. More specifically, these suicidal societies tended to be "altruistic" (in Durkheim's sense). That is, to be a member of the cult meant being willing to sacrifice oneself or die for the sake of a higher cause or good (reminiscent of Japanese officers committing *seppuku* in front of their troops after being defeated in World War II). Durkheim correctly observed that being socially integrated into some religious groups did not protect one against suicide because the norms of these religions (like the cults mentioned above) required self-sacrifice under many special circumstances. Thus, in Jonestown, the more social integration, the higher (not lower) the suicide rate.

Second, in most cults it is the charismatic leader's intentions that are crucial (e.g., Jim Jones, Adolf Hitler, David Koresh, etc.). Most cult leaders have a diffuse and extended concept of their own self. For example, both Jones and Koresh had sex with many women within their cults (and often forbade the women's own husbands from having sex with their wives) and sired many children. In a very real sense Jim Jones was the "father" of his cult and was in fact implanting his genes into cult members (in a sense magnifying or extending his "self"). It follows that for Jones or Koresh to kill "himself," he probably felt he also had to kill his extended family, that is, the entire cult. In this case the cult leader in effect decides for everyone else that they will "suicide." The leader's intentions or beliefs are paramount.

Third, there is usually perceived danger or persecution from the outside. Jones did not order the suicides until California Senator Leo Ryan came to Guyana to investigate the People's Temple. In Masada it was the Roman outsiders and in Waco it was the federal agents who seemed to trigger the suicides. Fourth, the cult tends to become isolated from the rest of larger society. Jones and his followers left California for Guyana and, ultimately, Guyana for heaven (or hell). This reminds us that all suicide is a transformation drive (cf. Hillman, 1964). That is, suicides want not so much to die as to *change themselves*, their lives, or their world (including going on to heaven or its equivalent). Routinely in cults the physical body is not held in very high regard. The soul or spirit is paramount and frequently it is maintained that one must renounce the physical body to get into heaven, or achieve *nirvana*, *moksha*, or religious transformation.

Finally, in almost all mass suicides there is coercion or even murder, especially of children or of the cult members who try to defect rather than suicide (or of wives and lovers by husbands in murder–suicides).

Although it is an overworked example of mass suicide, let us take a closer look at Jim Jones and the suicide in Guyana. Jones grew up in Indiana. His mother was an anthropologist who believed that her son eventually would become the messiah. Jones's father was a bigot, racist, and KKK member. Jones went to Butler University and was originally a Methodist minister. Later on Jones abandoned mainstream Christianity. Many of his earlier evangelical faith-healing "miracles" were in fact cheap tricks, such as producing chicken entrails when supposedly purging the ill of their cancers. Many members of the People's Temple were poor, relatively uneducated black African Americans who signed over the deeds to their homes or life insurance policies to Jim Jones. In California, family members began to protest to Senator Ryan about losing their property, money, and birth rights to Jones.

Partly to escape local ill-will, Jones fled to Guyana. There he and the cult became even more extremist. For example, Jones came to believe that the world would be destroyed by nuclear war. He grew increasingly paranoid. His cult lived in crowded conditions in temperatures often exceeding 100° Fahrenheit. Physical beatings, sexual abuse, and incest were commonplace in Jonestown. Jones practiced a form of terrorism in which children and spouses spied on family members and then told Jones, who chastized and severely punished (beat) the transgressors (as in Orwell's *1984*). Preparing for the end of the world, which he thought was imminent, Jones held drills or practices (called "white nights") in which cult members drank Kool-Aid, not knowing if it were poisoned – to prove their faith and loyalty to Jones. Note that all five of the traits of suicidal cults were present in Jones's People's Temple.

ORGANIZATIONAL SELF-DESTRUCTION

Another candidate for "social suicide" is organizational self-destruction. I remember in the 1960s, when I was a suicidology fellow, that my classmate at Johns Hopkins, Gene Brockhoff, had a goal of eliminating the Buffalo, New York, suicide prevention center, which he then directed. What ever happened to the Buffalo SPC, or to Gene Brockhoff for that matter? Before we can speculate on organizational suicide we have to have some idea of what the natural life expectancy of an organization is (Aldrich, 1979, reminds us that not all organizations are alike). Mayhew (1983) claims:

- Of 181 American automobile firms, 64% disappeared in less than 10 years.
- Of 10,000 business firms in Poughkeepsie, New York, 30% failed in one year; 78% failed in 10 years.
- The median life expectancy for small firms of less than 4 employees was 4 years.
- In general most business firms have a life expectancy about the same as a hound dog and just ahead of that of alley cats.

In a sense, organizations cannot "die" like individual human beings can. Organizations are not alive, conceived, or born, nor do they age in a strict biological connotation. For example, most businesses survive the deaths of their employees, even of a chief executive officer (CEO). Some organizations paradoxically seem to thrive by "killing" their employees, who are seen as replaceable.

I recently consulted on a cluster of executive suicides in a very large midwestern data-processing firm (this was a company with $4 billion in revenues in 1995). Six of their executives killed themselves in less than three months and another died in a small-plane crash. One of the key investigative questions was: Did the remarkable growth in this company contribute to or cause the suicides of its executives? The general perception in the employee interviews was "yes," it did. The company was seen as using up its employees by high stress, unrealistic expectations, long hours, and so forth; and then replacing them when they failed, got sick, or died (what the employees called an "Apache theory of management"). All that was seen to matter was the company profit (not individual well-being), as measured by an annual 20% growth rate and the company's latest stock values on the New York Stock Exchange. If employees did not concur with company work policies and growth objectives, they were let go. If they complied, then they often were worked to sickness or death. It turned out that the employees who could not "get with the program" were the suicides (although several had preexisting individual pathology). All the company suicides were either forced out (e.g., given sick leave), suspended, or fired; or blocked in promotion. In this company financial and social well-being for the firm was, in a real sense, perceived as being bought at the cost of individual suffering and even several suicides. Shades of Karl Marx!

Why do most organizations disappear? Historically there are two principal reasons: first, natural disasters (which are self-explanatory) and, second, social encounters. Mayhew (1983) argues that most organizations kill each other ("social homicide," if you will) through warfare or competition. But could an organization kill itself? Sure. An organization could:

- Declare bankruptcy
- Knowingly engage in excessive risk taking that leads to it own demise
- Deplete its resources (e.g., through embezzlement or poor management) such that it is unable to meet its obligations or is unable to fend off aggression from without or within

Although it seldom happens in very large companies, one could easily imagine reorganization via Chapter 11 bankruptcy proceedings to avoid excessive liabilities. Contemporary candidates would be Dow Corning to avoid liability for its silicone gel breast implants, Johns-Manville to avoid liabilities for the manufacture of cancer-related asbestos insulation, or the Ligget tobacco company to avoid the liabilities for sale and distribution of cigarettes. In such cases the corporation essentially destroys itself as it is presently organized to try to minimize liabilities, downsize, and then start over (a partial suicide?).

An interesting related business maneuver is something known in the corporate world as "suicide pill." A suicide pill is an automatic protective stock devaluing (of the company's treasury stocks) in the event of a hostile takeover attempt. By being prepared to devalue its own stocks, the company in effect is willing to kill itself to avoid a takeover. Knowing that such a procedure is in place theoretically discourages takeovers. Any company or individual that is willing to die gains great power over its competitors. Who in their right mind would want to take over a dead company?

Another example of organizational self-destruction would be a company or representative of an organization that engages in excessive or capricious risk taking that jeopardizes the life of the organization itself. One example is Ford Motor Company manufacturing the Ford Pinto automobile, knowing in advance that upon modest rear end collisions the gas tank could rupture and explode, burning the car's occupants (Maris, 1985). Ford and Lee Iacocca went ahead with the sale and distribution of the Pinto even though death and injury suits posed a substantial risk to the company (cf. the recent film "Class Action").

A second example is Adolf Hitler and Germany's behavior in World War II (see McRandle, *Track of the Wolf*, 1965). Hitler was a repeated failure who engaged in excessive risk taking for both himself and his country. For example, in 1900 Hitler failed math and natural history (in Realschule). Again, in 1905 he failed German (somewhat amusing, *nicht wahr*?)! By 1906 Hitler was so distraught that he decided "to end it all" by jumping in the Danube river. In 1909 Hitler failed to report for obligatory military service (another irony!). Later on in his political career the same failure and risk-taking behavior continued – only now it endangered the life of an entire nation. Crisis after crisis arose for Germany simply because Hitler failed to take action to prevent a predictable *bad* outcome. For example, Hitler made serious bad judgments in attacking Russia and in declaring war on the United States. By his choice of enemies, Adolf Hitler almost certainly assured his and Germany's defeat.

Third, and finally, attempts at personal gain by strategically placed employees or managers within a corporation could destroy the entire organization. Here we refer to individual profit taking by embezzlement, robbery, making unsecured loans, or financial speculation. Most organizations have built-in safeguards to prevent individuals from destroying the company or have sufficient resources such that the company could not be easily destroyed. Examples might include Ferdinand and Imelda Marcos's plundering of Filipino assets or recent losses by Lloyd's of London as a result of the financial indiscretions of a young Australian manager.

SOCIAL ANALOGUES TO INDIVIDUAL SUICIDES

Still another example of social suicide is when collectivity mimics or mirrors individual suicides. It is not too big a stretch of the imagination to conceive of industrial pollution as a kind of social overdose (Maris, 1971, p. 19; 1985, Chap. 14). One of the great paradoxes of Western urban–industrial development is that we are poisoning the air we breath, fouling the water that we drink, contaminating the soil in which our food and forests grow, and depleting unique, nonrenewable fossil and mineral resources. Today most of these industrial developments are "merely" life quality issues, not yet a social suicide for the Western world or the United States.

Consider some of the dimensions of America's social overdose. According to the Pollution Standard Index (a measure of five common pollutants; viz., sulfur dioxide, nitrogen dioxide, ozone, carbon monoxide, and solid particles in the air), the air in Los Angeles is unfit to breath for about two thirds of each year; and that in New York City, Chicago, Denver, and Pittsburgh is unfit to breath for one third of the year. When motor vehicles and industry operate, they produce sulfur dioxide and nitrogen oxide as emissions. As these emissions mix with water in the upper atmosphere, the result is sulfuric and nitric acid, which comes back to earth as acid rain – a kind of social overdose, if you will. Prevailing jet stream winds concentrate acid rain in the northeastern United States and in southeastern Canada. Acid rain kills hundreds of lakes and their fish (Adirondacks trout are so rare they are now probably worth about $200/lb), trees and forests on mountain tops (the acid destroys tree roots), and grasses and plants; and even destroys stone building surfaces.

Although the data are still unclear, there also seems to be a gradual global warming trend related to the "greenhouse effect." Escaping carbon dioxide acts like the glass on a greenhouse, reradiating heat escaping from the earth back to the earth. If the current warming trend continues, there could be a 3° to 6° Fahrenheit rise in world temperatures by the year 2050, which would melt ice caps and snow, flood some coastal cities, and alter the aquatic ecosystem.

One of the major pollutants is motor vehicle emissions. Cars, trucks, buses, and so forth, waste nonrenewable oil and gasoline, and produce nitrogen oxide and carbon monoxide as by-products. U.S. automobiles are the least fuel efficient cars in the world. If the U.S. "Big Three" automobile manufacturers raised the average car fuel economy to 40 miles per gallon, it would save as much energy as the country of Brazil consumes in an entire year. Detroit has workable carburetors that now get between 78 and 93 mpg; but they have not been put on the market for obvious economic reasons, not the least of which is the overlap in ownership of the oil and automobile industries and their greed for profit.

Another analogue to individual suicides and their use of firearms is the social proclivity for war, especially nuclear war. Not only is nuclear energy a dangerous carcinogen (one study in Denver, Colorado, found that those people who live downwind of the Rocky Flats Nuclear Weapons Plant had 24% more cancers than those living upwind, controlling for other factors), an all-out nuclear war cannot be won and must never be fought. The ultimate act of violence is a full-blown international nuclear war, a war that could destroy life itself. At least when individuals suicide, life continues. The survivors (*hibakusha*) of the A-bombs in Hiroshima and Nagasaki, Japan, in 1945 were afraid that nature herself had been poisoned, that the flowers and trees would not bloom again next Spring. Nuclear death is mega-death, the potential of the loss of continuity of generations, even of history – total annihilation.

Social suicide is a real prospect when psychotic leaders (like Libya's Khadafy) have nuclear weapons. Too many countries who do not get along (e.g., have fundamental racial, religious, or ethnic differences) now have nuclear weapons (viz., USA, China, the former Soviet Union, Britain, France, Israel, South Africa, Argentina, Brazil, Pakistan, etc.). A major nuclear war is an unthinkable psychotic nightmare. Assuming about 5000 megatons of nuclear warheads were detonated: (1) it would be pitch black initially in the target zones; (2) the sun-blocking smog would be highly radioactive for a very long time (if the initial blast did not kill immediately, survivors would suffer hemorrhaging, diarrhea, lesions, anemia, immunological damage, pneumonia, and gastroenterological disorders); (3) it would become very cold (e.g., 0° –20° Fahrenheit in July in the U.S.) – most living creatures including plants would literally freeze to death; and (4) there would be droughts and fierce storms at sea. At least one half of the world's population would die as a result of such a nuclear holocaust. And the irony is that we would have done it to ourselves under the guise of deterrence, a social suicide for over half the world's population.

MILITARY SUICIDES

Historically, the first (540 B.C.) artistic reference (on a vase) was to the Greek soldier Ajax falling on his sword after defeat in battle, as did Saul and his sword bearer in the Hebrew bible. Military suicides tend to be one of two types. In the first type, the original aggression is external to one's self but gets retroflexed if the battle is lost. This is clearly a social suicide because, if social events were different (e.g., if you defeated your enemy), then your suicide would not be necessary. Note that here, suicide is not much different from homicide, in that the underlying motivation is to kill someone. Further, defeat-in-battle suicides suggest either unexpended aggressive energy (as in some murder–suicides) that gets turned back on one's self or that the ultimate act of external aggression is to rob your enemy of control of a defeated victim (as has been suggested in the suicide of Adolf Hitler). Here suicide is a kind of victory even in defeat – killing one's self to prevent others from having the pleasure of executing you or of demonstrating their power over you. As with rape, military suicide is sometimes more about power than about sex or death.

Second, military suicide is often altruistic suicide. For example, young *kamikaze* pilots in World War II were dying for the Emperor and for the greater good of Japan. The same is probably true for Muslims who strap bombs to themselves and blow up buses in Jerusalem; that is, the death is for Allah. Such military suicides are self-sacrifices intended to bring about social, political, or religious change. Thus, altruistic suicides are obligatory deaths in the interests of a presumed larger social good, like a mother sacrificing herself to save her child and its future.

A related altruistic suicide type is illustrated among the Yuit Eskimos of St. Lawrence Island, as described by Leighton and Hughes (see Maris, 1981, p. 238 ff.). The Yuit are a hunting and gathering society. If the husband asks his family three times to allow him to suicide, his wife and children are obligated either to shoot or hang him (i.e., an assisted suicide). Such altruistic suicide often occurs when the husband is ill or injured and has become a liability to the welfare or even survival of the tribe or family (e.g., he can no longer hunt or travel). Among the Yuit, suicide is not stigmatized in such circumstances. In fact this suicide is seen as courageous and rational. Before the suicide the victim dresses as if he were already dead (e.g., turns his fur parka inside out, with the hair touching his skin) and then walks to the destroying place. The victim tells the survivors that they are able to take care of themselves now, to respect the elderly, and gives a brief statement about their philosophy of life. Then the wife either shoots her husband or several relatives help hang the victim. Usually a period of isolation and purification follows for those participating in the suicide.

Sometimes suicide is social because it involves risk taking and contingencies. For example, among the Tikopia (Firth, 1961) young women usually swim out to sea and young men put out to sea in a canoe in their suicide attempts. If the community's response to a suicide attempt is vigorous and prompt, and the would-be suicide is rescued, then all is forgiven and the suicide attempter is reintegrated into Tikopian society. On the other hand, if the group's response is not very enthusiastic or prompt (which may say something about how the group feels about the would-be suicide), often the attempt will succeed.

CONCLUSIONS

Of course, we could continue to examine other candidates for social suicide. Clearly, a suicide pact has social overtones and dynamics (Wickett, 1989), as do suicides that are witnessed by other people (McDowell, Rothberg, & Koshes, 1994). However, we now start to become redundant. To conclude: at first blush suicide seems like the ultimate private action because the individual's mind and intentions are a defining trait of the suicide. But suicide is also eminently public and social. Suicides result because of social forces and pathologies acting in concert with individual characteristics. We have seen that some suicides are committed to preserve society, not to weaken it. Thus, ultimately, if we wish to prevent suicide or lower suicide rates, then we need to see suicide as a social act. As such, suicide prevention requires social, economic, and cultural transformations at the primary prevention level—not just individual counseling and dispensing of the latest antidepressants.

REFERENCES

Aldrich, H. E. (1979). *Organizations and environments.* Englewood Cliffs, NJ: Prentice-Hall.

Berman, A. L., & Jobes D. A. (1991). *Adolescent suicide.* Washington, DC: American Psychological Press.

Durkheim, E. (1938). *The Rules of Sociological Method.* Glencoe, IL: Free Press. (Original work published 1895)

Durkheim, E. (1951). *Suicide.* Glencoe, IL: Free Press. (Original work published 1897)

Firth, R. (1961). Suicide and risk-taking in Tikopia society. *Psychiatry, 24,* 2–17.

Hillman, J. (1964). *Suicide and the soul.* New York: Harper & Row.

Maris, R. W. (1971). Social suicide. In D. B. Anderson and L. J. McLean (Eds.), *Identifying suicide potential* (pp. 15–20). New York: Behavioral Publications.

Maris, R. W. (1981). *Pathways to suicide.* Baltimore: Johns Hopkins.

Maris, R. W. (1985). *Social problems.* Belmont, CA: Wadsworth.

Maris, R. W. (1989). The social relations of suicide. In D. J. Jacobs and H. N. Brown (Eds.), *Suicide: Understanding and Responding* (pp. 87–125). Madison, CT: International Universities Press.

Maris, R. W. (1992). Suicide. In E. F. Borgatta and M. I. Borgatta (Eds.), *Encyclopedia of sociology* (Vol. 4, pp. 2111–2119). New York: Macmillian.

Maris, R. W. (1996). Suicide. In R. Dulbecco (Ed.), *Encyclopedia of human biology* (Vol. 7). San Diego, CA: Academic Press.

Martindale, D. (1981). *The nature and types of sociological theory.* Boston: Houghton-Mifflin.

Mayhew, B. H. (1983). Hierarchical differentiation in imperatively coordinated associations. In *Re-*

search in the sociology of organizations (Vol. 2, pp. 153–229). JAI Press.
McDowell, C. P., Rothberg, J. M., & Koshes, R. J. (1994). Witnessed suicides. *Suicide and Life-Threatening Behavior, 24*(3), 213–223.
McRandle, J. H. (1965). *Track of the wolf.* Evanston, IL: Northwestern University.
Wickett, A. (1989). *Double-exit.* Eugene, OR: Hemlock Society.
Wittgenstein, L. (1953). *Philosophical investigations.* New York: Macmillian.
Wolff, K. H. (Ed.). (1950). *The sociology of Georg Simmel.* Glencoe, IL: Free Press.

PART II. Cultural Perspectives

6
Suicide in America: A Nation of Immigrants

David Lester

The patterns of suicide of immigrants are briefly explored, followed by a more detailed study of the suicidal behavior of Chinese in different nations of the world (including America), African American slaves in the 1600s and 1700s, and Native Americans. Some of the implications of the issues addressed are explored for their relevance in counseling clients from different cultures.

A cursory glance at recent suicide statistics in America reveals that the suicide rate has remained remarkably constant over the last 20 years – mostly around 12 per 100,000 per year. Indeed, since 1945 the rate has ranged only from 9.8 to 13.3. In contrast, other nations of the world have witnessed dramatic increases in their suicide rate during this period (nations such as Norway, from 6.5 to 16.8) or decreases (such as England and Wales, from 12.1 to 7.4).

If we look more closely at the American suicide rate, we do find differences by gender, with male suicide rates increasing in recent years and female suicide rates decreasing, and we also can find differences by age. But the theme of this volume focuses on cultural and international perspectives, and so I would like to focus on the ethnic and cultural differences in patterns of suicide in the United States. As the title of my paper indicates, the U.S. is a nation of relatively recent immigrants and the descendants of immigrants – and the patterns of suicidal behavior in the different ethnic groups differ greatly and raise some fascinating issues.

SUICIDE IN IMMIGRANT GROUPS

Many years ago, Sainsbury and Barraclough (1968) correlated the suicide rates of 11 nations in 1959 with the suicide rates of immigrants from those nations to America and found a strong association, despite the fact that the suicide rates for the immigrant groups were on the whole higher than the suicide rates of those who remained in their home nations. Immigration is perhaps stressful (or perhaps the more suicidal people decide to emigrate), but, for example, the Irish had one of the lowest suicide rates of the nations studied in 1959 and Irish immigrants were one of the groups with the lowest suicide rates among the immigrant groups (Dublin, 1963).[1] This general result has been replicated in Australia (Burvill, Woodings, Stenhouse, and McCall, 1982; Lester, 1972, 1980; Sainsbury, 1973), Canada (Kliewer & Ward, 1988), and America as a whole (Lester, 1980); and also in Chicago in the 1920s (Lester, 1989a). Immigrants come from a particular culture and bring their culture with them when they emigrate, a culture that involves language, dress, codes of behavior, and perhaps the risk of suicidal behavior. Interestingly, however, Burvill et al. (Burvill, McCall,

[1]Incidentally, these results provide evidence for the relative reliability and validity of national suicide rates despite the differences among nations in the methods for certifying the cause of death.

David Lester is with the Center for the Study of Suicide, RR41, 5 Stonegate Court, Blackwood, NJ 08012.

Suicide and Life-Threatening Behavior, Vol. 27(1), Spring 1997

Reid, & Stenhouse, 1973; Burvill, McCall, Woodings, & Stenhouse, 1983) noted that British immigrants to Australia quickly changed their methods for committing suicide once they arrived in Australia, suggesting that the availability of methods for suicide may be important in this choice (Clarke & Lester, 1989).

Suicidal behavior may be quite differently determined and have different meanings in different cultures. The classic study demonstrating this was Hendin's (1964) study of suicide in Scandinavia. In Denmark, Danish mothers created strong dependency in their sons which led to depression and suicidality after adult experiences of loss or separation. In Sweden, there was a strong emphasis on performance and success by parents, resulting in ambitious children for whom work was central to their lives. Suicide typically followed failure in performance that had damaged the men's self-esteem. In Norway, where the suicide rate was lower, there was strong dependency of the sons on their mothers, but Norwegian children were less passive and more aggressive than Danish children. Alcohol abuse was more common, and Norwegian men were more open about their feelings – able to laugh at themselves and cry more openly. These national patterns will probably continue to have influence on the immigrants from these nations in America.

Lester (1987) proposed a social deviancy theory of suicide in which groups that found themselves deviant from the community in social characteristics would experience more stress and, as a result, exhibit more psychiatric disorder and suicidal behavior. Consistent with this theory, Lester found that, the smaller the size of an immigrant group in Australia, the higher the suicide rate of that group, but he failed to replicate this finding in Canada (Lester, 1986, 1987, 1994d).

This is the general pattern for immigrants, but let us look at one immigrant group to America in particular, Chinese Americans, a group of interest because the Chinese are native to many nations (such as the People's Republic of China and Hong Kong) and have emigrated in large numbers to nations such as America.

SUICIDE IN CHINESE

The suicide rates of Asian Americans are relatively low compared to Whites in America. For example, in 1980 in America, the suicide rates were 13.3 per 100,000 per year for Native Americans, 13.2 for white Americans, 9.1 for Japanese Americans, 8.3 for Chinese Americans, 6.1 for African Americans, and 3.5 for Filipino Americans (Lester, 1994a).

Lester noted that the patterns of suicide also differed for these ethnic groups. The ratio of the male to female suicide rates was much larger for Whites and African Americans than for Asian Americans, and whereas suicide rates increased with age for Asian Americans, the suicide rates peaked in young adulthood for African Americans and Native Americans. Asian Americans used hanging for suicide much more often than Whites and African Americans, and used firearms relatively less often.

Lester concluded that the epidemiology of Asian Americans in America showed similarities to the results of epidemiological studies of Asian Americans in their home nations, indicating that cultural factors have an important influence on the circumstances of suicidal behavior.

Lester (1994b) then examined the epidemiology of suicide in Chinese in Hong Kong, Singapore, Taiwan, the People's Republic of China, Hawaii, and the United States as a whole. A couple of examples here will illustrate the results. The ratio of the male to female suicide rates in 1980 was 1.2 for Chinese Americans, 1.2 for Hong Kong residents, 1.2 for Taiwanese residents, and 1.2 for Singapore Chinese, identical gender ratios. Suicide rates peaked in the elderly in all the nations: for those 65 and older in Chinese Americans, 75 and older in Hong Kong and Taiwan, and 70 and older in Singapore Chinese – the nations used different classifications by age.

As suggested by Burvill et al. (1983), the methods used for suicide did differ for the different groups of Chinese: jumping was more common in Singapore and Hong Kong, hanging in Chinese Americans, and poisons in Taiwan, probably a result of the difference between the nations in the availability of methods for suicide. For example, Lester (1994c) showed that the use of jumping for suicide in Singapore was strongly associated with the development of high-rise apartments. Furthermore, the suicide rates differed: in 1980 the rates were 13.5 in Singapore Chinese and Hong Kong, 10.0 in Taiwan, and 8.3 for Chinese Americans.

Thus, gender and age patterns in Chinese suicide seem to be affected strongly by ethnicity, whereas the absolute suicide rates and methods used are affected by the nation in which the Chinese dwell.

SUICIDE IN AFRICAN AMERICAN SLAVES

Of course, not all immigrant Americans came here freely as a result of their own decisions. Many were brought here as slaves. When I visited the National Civil Rights Museum in Memphis, Tennessee, a few years ago, I noticed that the exhibit for 1619 mentioned that slaves fought against their bondage by stealing, escape, arson, and as a last resort, suicide. This motivated me to explore suicide in the enslaved in greater depth (Lester, 1996a); let me review a few of my findings here.

Suicide was very common among the slaves when they were captured, while they were being transported to America, and immediately upon arrival (Piersen, 1977). The myth was widespread in Africa that Whites cooked and ate the captured Africans, and the slave traders helped perpetuate the myth—the English traders claiming that the Portuguese traders did eat their victims and vice versa. Slaves watching Whites drink red wine often thought that they were drinking blood (du Pratz, 1763). Slaves already in America, helping to deal with the newly arrived slaves, also teased the newcomers with these stories. As a result, some slaves did commit suicide to escape being eaten, and mass suicides were not uncommon. Snelgrave (1734) reported groups of more than 20 slaves hanging themselves in the West Indies. Nobility, older slaves, and male slaves seemed to fare worse, and Ibo slaves from Nigeria were noted for their high rate of suicide. Many African tribes believed that the soul returned home after death, and so suicide was seen by some as a means of returning to their homelands.

Ellenberger (1960), in writing of the involuntary commitment of psychiatric patients and of wild animals captured for zoos, noted that the trauma of captivity can be severe, leading to two syndromes—anxiety and self-mutilation or depression and stupor—and Piersen noted that the slaves often showed these syndromes on the slave ships and after arrival.

Commentators disagree how common suicide was among the those born into slavery, but statistical data are lacking for the early years. However, I located mortality data for 1850 that enabled me to calculate suicide rates by ethnic group (Lester, 1966a). I calculated the suicide rate for Whites as 2.12 per 100,000 per year, for Black slaves 0.72, and for freed Black slaves 1.15.[2] The rates follow the same pattern for both males and females.

Although, of course, these statistics may be quite unreliable, for even contemporary suicide statistics are criticized for inaccuracies, it is interesting to note that the ethnic difference here is found currently in America, where Whites have higher suicide rates than African Americans (Lester, 1994a), and in African nations such as Zimbabwe and South Africa (Lester, 1989b; Lester & Wilson, 1988).

The possible phenomenon of high suicide rates during capture and transportation combined with lower suicide rates later has modern parallels. Kwiet (1984) noted that the suicide rate was high among

[2]The source for the statistics classifies African Americans as Blacks and Mulattos.

Jews in Austria during the period of rounding up by the Nazis and transportation to the concentration camps, but lower later in the camps. The uncertainty about the future may later be replaced by clear external agents to blame for one's misery, and perhaps anger develops to compete with anxiety and depression, a situation that Henry and Short (1954) in their theory of suicide and homicide viewed as decreasing the risk of suicide.

Under what circumstances did the enslaved commit suicide? I found examples of suicide in slaves after severe punishment, after unsuccessful rebellion, and when threatened with separation from a spouse and children as a result of being sold to another slave owner.

Why was suicide not more common among the enslaved? Initially, the slave owners tried to deter suicide by mutilating the corpses, hoping that the slaves would be deterred from committing suicide in order to return to their homeland if their bodies were dismembered. As the slaves adopted the Christian religion, suicides were branded as criminals and denied Christian burial. Today, the African American church is strongly opposed to suicide (Early, 1992), and the view of suicide as acceptable only as a very last resort in the face of extreme stress is consistent with modern Afrocentric optimal psychology (e.g., Myers, 1993).

SUICIDE IN NATIVE AMERICANS[3]

When the immigrants, voluntary and forced, arrived in America, they found, of course, an earlier group of immigrants, who perhaps migrated from Asia across from what is now Russia into Alaska and down through the Americas some 12 to 15 thousand years ago – Native Americans. Much has been written in recent years about suicidal behavior in Native Americans, and here I address only two issues: first, is the high rate of suicide sometimes found in groups of Native Americans a new phenomenon or have these groups always had high suicide rates, and secondly, what is the role of the clash of cultures in precipitating suicide in Native Americans?

Suicide in the Past

Jilek-Aall (1988) noted that suicide was present in traditional Native American societies, among the elderly and infirm, to prevent capture in warfare, or as atonement. Suicides in the past were often honored. Youths today learn this from the stories told by their elders, and perhaps today's youth hope for attention and acceptance in their own suicides.

I am engaged in a project tracking down reports of suicidal behavior in Native American tribes from previous centuries to see whether suicidal behavior occurred and under what circumstances. Let me briefly report some of the earliest occurrences that I have found so far.

Wallace (1972) has reprinted accounts by a visitor to the Iroquois in the 1600s.

> "Some Savages," reported LeMercier of the Huron, "told us that one of the principal reasons why they showed so much indulgence toward their children, was that when the children saw themselves treated by their parents with some severity, they usually resorted to extreme measures and hanged themselves, or ate of a certain root they call *Audachienrra*, which is a very quick poison." . . . while suicides by frustrated children were not actually frequent, there are nevertheless a number of recorded cases of suicide where parental interference was the avowed cause. (pp. 38–39)

Le Clercq (1910) reported on the Micmac for the period 1675 to 1686.

> The Gaspesians, however, are so sensitive to affronts which are offered them that they sometimes abandon themselves to despair, and even make attempts on their own lives, in the belief that the insult which has been done them tarnishes the honour and the reputation which they have acquired, whether in war or in hunting. (p. 247)

He gave the account of a boy who, having been inadvertently hit by a servant, went

[3]This section is based on Lester (1996b).

out and hung himself from a tree, only to be rescued by his sister, who was passing by. His brother had earlier hung himself because he was refused by a girl whom he loved and whom he wanted to marry. The women and girls tended to commit suicide more often as a result of grief after the death of their relatives and friends, typically by hanging also.

Writing of the Delaware, Heckewelder (1819) noted that they saw suicide as a result of mental disorder.

> Between the years 1771 and 1780, four Indians on my acquaintance took the root of may-apple, which is commonly used on such occasions, in order to poison themselves, in which they all succeeded, except one. Two of them were young men, who had been disappointed in love, the girls on whom they had fixed their choice, and to whom they were engaged, having changed their minds and married other lovers. (p. 251)

One of the remaining cases was a married man whose wife took a lover, and he was depressed at the thought of having to leave her and his children. He had hoped that the lover would not follow them when they went to their sugar camp, but he came home from work one day to find the lover with his wife. He left the camp and killed himself by eating a poisonous root.

Zeisberger (1910), writing about the Delaware in the period of 1767 to 1780, also reported that suicide was not uncommon among the men if they discovered their wives to have been unfaithful.

> Many a one takes her unfaithfulness so to heart that in the height of his despair he swallows a poisonous root, which generally causes death in two hours, unless an antidote be administered in good time: this is often done, the Indians knowing that the properties of certain herbs counteract each other and being able to judge from the effects what poison has been taken. Women, also, have been known to destroy themselves on account of a husband's unfaithfulness. (p. 83)

Of course, we do not have many of these accounts, and we cannot estimate suicide rates from the reports. But the accounts are of interest because they come from an era when the clash of the two cultures was in its early stages.

The Clash of Cultures

The conflict between the traditional Native American culture and the dominant American culture has often been viewed as providing a major role in precipitating Native American suicide. May and Dizmang (1974) noted that three major sociological theories have been proposed for explaining the Native American suicide rate. One theory focuses on *social disorganization.* The dominance of the Anglo-American culture has forced Native American culture to change and has eroded traditional cultural systems and values. This changes the level of social regulation and social integration, important causal factors for suicide in Durkheim's (1897) theory of suicide.

A second theory focuses on *cultural conflict* itself. The pressure, especially from the educational system and mass media, on Native Americans, especially the youth, to acculturate, a pressure that is opposed by their elders, leads to great stress for the youths.

A third theory focuses on the *breakdown of the family* in Native American tribes. Parents are often unemployed, substance abusers, and in trouble with the law, and divorce and desertion of the family by one or more parents is common.

Acculturation occurs when a culture encounters a dominant alternative culture. The resulting pressure from the dominant culture leads to a variety of changes in the nondominant culture (Berry, 1990): physical changes (such as type of housing, urbanization, and increasing population density), biological changes (resulting from changing diet and exposure to new diseases), political changes (such as loss of autonomy for the nondominant culture), economic changes (such as changes in type of employment), cultural changes (in language, religion, education, and the arts), social relationships (both within the culture and between the two cultures), and psychological changes at the individual level (in behavior, values, attitudes, and motives).

Berry noted that four possibilities are

open to the nondominant culture: *integration* – maintaining relations with the dominant culture while maintaining cultural identity; *assimilation* – maintaining relations with the dominant culture but not maintaining cultural identity; *separation* – not maintaining relations with the dominant culture but maintaining cultural identity; and *marginalization* – not maintaining relations with the dominant culture and not maintaining cultural identity.

It would be of great interest to categorize the different Native American tribes as to which strategy appears to have been chosen and to examine the different consequences for the society and for the individuals in the society.

Does Cultural Conflict Cause Suicide?

Although the problem of acculturation has been proposed as one of the major causes of depression and suicidal behavior among Native Americans, the majority of research reports on Native American individuals who attempt or complete suicide mention precipitating causes such as grief over loss, quarrels with relatives and friends, and so forth. Rarely is cultural conflict listed among the precipitating causes. Of course, it may be that the problems of acculturation raise the stress level of individuals so much that stressors, which under ordinary circumstances would not precipitate suicide, now do so.

A few brief case histories have been published that illustrate the problems of acculturation and culture conflict. For example, Berlin (1986) described the case of a bright young Native American woman who completed undergraduate school and qualified as a teacher, and who was admitted to graduate school. Her clan, however, told her that she was required to teach on the Reservation. Her desire to go to graduate school was seen as striving to be better than her peers, and this was unacceptable and forbidden. The young woman had a psychiatric breakdown and was hospitalized. In a similar situation, the tribe and another family could not decide whether to let a young woman go to graduate school for an MBA after she obtained her undergraduate degree and, during the long wait for a decision, she attempted suicide.

In this latter case, the young woman, whom Berlin called Josie, had alcoholic parents who frequently sent her and her brothers and sisters to live with relatives while they went on drinking sprees. A teacher realized Josie's potential and received permission for Josie to live with her. With this teacher's help, her academic performance improved, and she went to college. Josie now resented that her parents, who had neglected her, were involved in decisions about her life. The clan leadership and tribal council were relatively enlightened about the issues and eventually gave permission for Josie to attend graduate school. While at graduate school, Josie underwent psychotherapy to deal with her depression and anger, and other personal problems. After graduation, she returned to the tribe to manage their business office, marrying a young man who had fought a similar battle in order to obtain an MSW degree.

On the other hand, Westermeyer (1979) provided cases of Native Americans seen at the University of Minnesota Hospitals for whom trying to live in the mainstream American culture had presented problems. Westermeyer felt that identity problems were perhaps no more common in Native Americans than in Whites, but that Native Americans did show a unique type of identity problem, namely, ambivalent or negative feelings about their ethnic identity. Westermeyer presented urban Native Americans who illustrate this problem.

Five of the patients, ranging in age from 12 to 23, had identity crises – they experienced conflict about their Native American identity and about what being "Indian" meant. All were students and economically dependent upon others. For example, one young girl, who was seen after a suicide attempt, had her Indian mother die two years earlier. She then lived with her White father and six siblings for a year. The father had trouble supporting them and sent the children to live with their Indian maternal grandmother. The patient began to use drugs and to have problems with her White teachers at school. Eventually a White welfare worker sent her to a White foster home, at which point she attempted suicide. In the hospital, she said, "I'm the only Indian here and I hate everybody like they hate me." She had a recurrent dream in which she gave birth to a baby girl with blue eyes whom she loved but whom she also wanted to injure.

In the five adolescents, Westermeyer noted two different types of problems. The two boys were raised to assume a White middle-class identity but found this difficult because of their physical characteristics. The three girls were raised by Indian mothers who had rejected being Indian. Loss of their mothers, together with abandonment by their White fathers, led to anger. Their problems were made worse by social workers placing them in White foster homes.

Five of the cases were judged to have a negative identity. These were older than the patients with identity crises, and all were male. They were estranged from their Indian family members, and they lived as lower-class individuals on the periphery of the White society. One patient was admitted with hallucinations and paranoid delusions after a drinking binge. He had a record of multiple psychiatric admissions. Although he supported the idea of Indian activism, he felt estranged from Indians, had little respect for them, and avoided them. He had joined a Jewish student activist group that he admired, and he wondered whether his Indian tribe might be a lost tribe of Israel. He identified himself as a Zionist.

Research on Acculturation

Bagley (1991) looked at the suicide rate of Canadian Indian males aged 15 to 34 on the 26 most populated Reservations in Alberta, Canada, and found that the more isolated reservations had the higher suicide rates. In contrast, Garro (1988) found that the suicide rates in the more isolated communities in Manitoba were lower than in the more accessible communities. Thus, these Canadian results appear to be in conflict.

Bachman (1992) examined the correlates of the suicide rate in 120 counties in America that are partially or totally located on Reservation land and found that economic deprivation, rather than acculturation, seemed to be the strongest correlate of Native American suicide rates.

Supportive results for the influence of acculturation on suicide in Native Americans comes from Van Winkle and May (1986), who examined suicide rates in three groups of Native Americans in New Mexico (the Apache, Navajo, and Pueblo) and attempted to account for the differences in terms of the degree of acculturation. Overall, the crude suicide rates were 43.3 per 100,000 for the Apache, 27.8 for the Pueblo, and 12.0 for the Navajo.

The Jicarilla and Mescalero Apache of New Mexico were originally nomadic hunters and gatherers, organized into self-sufficient bands whose leaders held limited power. Their religion had no organized priesthood and was not a cohesive force in their lives. Individualism was a highly valued characteristic. Today they live in homes scattered about the Reservation or in border towns. They raise livestock, cut timber, or work in tribally owned businesses. Formal tribal governments have been established, but religion remains unimportant. Individualism is still valued. However, the raiding parties that formerly provided a some degree of social integration have been eliminated. The Apache appear, therefore, to have few integrating forces in their culture, and Van Winkle and May saw their high suicide rate as a direct result of this lack of integration.

The Apache have been in contact with Whites quite intensely. Their Reservations are small and surrounded by White communities. Indeed many Apache live in mixed communities. Thus, the Apache have low social integration and high acculturation.

The Pueblo traditionally lived in compact towns and engaged in agriculture. Religion permeated their lives and was a strong integrating force. There was an organized priesthood and religious societies that took care of religious and civil matters. Individualism was discouraged and conformity valued. Thus, the Pueblo were the most integrated group, and Van Winkle and May found their intermediate suicide rate a puzzle. They tried to explain the Pueblo having the second highest suicide rate using the concept of acculturation. The Pueblo have had increasing contact with Whites since 1959. Many of the Pueblos are near large cities such as Albuquerque and Santa Fe. Thus, they have high social integration and moderate but increasing acculturation. For the larger Pueblo tribes, Van Winkle and May compared the suicide rates of those tribes that had acculturated and those that had remained traditional, and found a clear tendency for the acculturated and transitional tribes to have the higher suicide rates.

The Navajo, who have the lowest suicide rate, were nomadic hunters and gatherers who later settled down and turned to agriculture. They are organized into bands, but matrilineal clans exert a strong influence. Although religion is important in their lives, they have no organized priesthood. Individualism is valued but not as strongly as among the Apache. Thus, their social integration appears to be intermediate between that of the Apache and that of the Pueblo. However, the Navajo had been the most geographically and socially isolated from Whites of the three groups until the 1970s, when mineral exploration increased on their reservations and some Navajo began to take wage-earning jobs.

Van Winkle and May's explanation of the suicide rates in the three groups can be summarized as shown in Table 1. It can be seen that acculturation performed better than social integration an as explanation of the differing suicide rates in these three tribes.

Counseling and Culture

It may be asked whether there are implications of this for counseling and psychotherapy. It is sometimes argued that only "like" can counsel "like"; that is, that only homosexuals can counsel homosexuals, women counsel women, ex-addicts counsel addicts, and so on. Is the same true also for different cultures? The majority of counselors and psychotherapists deny this, claiming that a good counselor or psychotherapist can counsel any kind of patient. However, to counsel someone very different in background from oneself may require that the counselor learn about the background and culture from which the individual comes.

Connors (1996), a Native Canadian, has presented the case of Robin, a 13-year-old Ojibway boy, adopted by White parents when he was 2 years old. From the time of his adoption, Robin had shown a great deal of anger and difficulty in forming healthy emotional attachments. He had destroyed property, set fire to the house, and killed a pet. In his teenage years, he

TABLE 1

	Social Integration	Acculturation	Suicide Rate
Apache	Low	High	High
Pueblo	High	Moderate	Moderate
Navajo	Moderate	Low	Low

lied, stole, and used drugs. Connors recognized that these problems stemmed from his separation from and abandonment by his biological parents, and that Robin felt alienated from the White culture into which he had been transferred.

Connors recommended that Robin join an Ojibway Adolescent Treatment Program. He was reintroduced to Ojibway cultural ways and received counseling from an Ojibway counselor. He joined an Ojibway drum group and learned to sing in Ojibway and to dance Pow Wow. After some time in the program, he decided to go and live with his Ojibway extended family, and his counselors helped him make contact with them and move back. Connors continued to counsel him, and Robin's anger and self-destructive behavior soon disappeared.

Sue and Sue (1990) presented the case of Janet, a Chinese-American female college senior majoring in sociology, who came to the college counseling center complaining of depression, feelings of worthlessness, and suicidal thoughts. She had difficulty identifying the causes of her depression, but she seemed quite hostile to the psychotherapist, who was also Chinese American.

Discussion of this revealed that Janet resented being seen by a Chinese psychotherapist, feeling that she had been assigned to one because of her own race. Janet disliked everything Chinese, including Chinese men, whom she found sexually unattractive. She dated only White men, which had upset her parents. However, her last romance had broken up partly because her boyfriend's parents objected to him dating a Chinese woman.

Janet clearly had difficulties in her continuing denial of her Chinese heritage. She was being forced to realize that she was Chinese, for she was not fully accepted by White America. Initially she blamed the Chinese for her dilemma, but then she turned her hostility toward herself. Feeling alienated from her own culture and rejected by the White culture, she was experiencing an identity crisis with a resulting depression.

The psychotherapist in such a case must deal with cultural racism and its effects on minorities. Positive acculturation must be distinguished from rejection of one's own cultural values, as well as typical adolescent rebellion from one's parents. Psychotherapists can work with such a client more effectively if they are conversant with the cultural history and experiences of their clients.

DISCUSSION

By focusing on the suicidal behavior of different ethnic groups in America, we can easily see the strong influence of the culture upon the individual; and we can also see the role that culture conflict and acculturation plays in affecting the rate, the meaning of, and the circumstances of suicidal behavior.

However, acculturation does not always lead to an increased incidence of suicide (or other disturbed behaviors). Social scientists should work on identifying which cultural characteristics enable some cultures to acculturate with few social and personal problems while other cultures develop many problems. Counselors should take into account the cultures from which their clients come and the type of acculturation problems that their clients face; and counselors should help clients decide whether and the extent to which they want to acculturate and facilitate the client's choice, whatever it might be.

REFERENCES

Bachman, R. (1992). *Death and violence on the reservation.* New York: Auburn House.

Bagley, C. (1991). Poverty and suicide among Native Canadians. *Psychological Reports, 69,* 149–150.

Berlin, I. N. (1986). Psychopathology and its antecedents among American Indian adolescents. *Advances in Clinical Child Psychology, 9,* 125–152.

Berry, J. W. (1990). Acculturation and adaptation. *Arctic Medical Research, 49.* 142–150.

Burvill, P., McCall, M., Reid, T., & Stenhouse, N. (1973). Methods of suicide of English and Welsh immigrants in Australia. *British Journal of Psychiatry, 123,* 285–294.

Burvill, P., McCall, M., Woodings, T., & Stenhouse, N. (1983). Comparison of suicide rates and methods in English, Scots and Irish immigrants in Australia. *Social Science and Medicine, 17*, 705-708.

Burvill, P., Woodings, T., Stenhouse, N., & McCall, M. (1982). Suicide during 1961-1970 in migrants in Australia. *Psychological Medicine, 12*, 295-308.

Clarke, R. V., & Lester, D. (1989). *Suicide: Closing the exits.* New York: Springer-Verlag.

Connors, E. A. (1996, in press). The healing path. In A. A. Leenaars & D. Lester (Eds.), *Suicide and the unconscious.* Northvale, NJ: Jason Aronson.

Dublin, L. I. (1963). *Suicide.* New York: Ronald Press.

Du Pratz, L. P. (1763). *The history of Louisiana.* London, Becket and P. A. de Hondt.

Durkheim, E. (1897). *Le suicide.* Paris: Felix Alcan.

Early, K. E. (1992). *Religion and suicide in the African-American community.* Westport, CT: Greenwood.

Ellenberger, E. (1960). Zoological garden and mental hospital. *Canadian Psychiatric Association Journal, 5*, 136-149.

Garro, L. C. (1988). Suicides by status Indians in Manitoba. *Arctic Medical Research, 47*(Suppl. 1), 590-592.

Heckewelder, J. (1819). An account of the history, manners and customs of the Indian nations who once inhabited Pennsylvania and neighboring states. *Transactions of the Historical and Literary Committee of the American Philosophical Society, 1*(1), 1-348.

Hendin, H. (1964). *Suicide and Scandinavia.* New York: Grune & Stratton.

Henry, A. F., & Short, J. F. (1954). *Suicide and homicide.* Glencoe, IL: Free Press.

Jilek-Aall, L. (1988). Suicidal behavior among youth. *Transcultural Psychiatric Research Review, 29*(2), 87-105.

Kliewer, E. V., & Ward, R. H. (1988). Convergence of immigrant suicide rates to those in the destination country. *American Journal of Epidemiology, 127*, 640-653.

Kwiet, K. (1984). The ultimate refuge. *Leo Baeck Institute Yearbook, 29*, 135-167.

Le Clercq, C. (1910). *New relation of Gaspesia.* Toronto: Champlain Society.

Lester, D. (1972). Migration and suicide. *Medical Journal of Australia, 1*, 941-942.

Lester, D. (1980). The validity of national suicide rates. *British Journal of Psychiatry, 136*, 107-108.

Lester, D. (1986). Suicide rates in immigrants to Australia. *Medical Journal of Australia, 144*, 280.

Lester, D. (1987). Social deviancy and suicide. *Journal of Social Psychology, 127*, 339-340.

Lester, D. (1989a). Suicide rates in immigrant groups and their countries of origin. *Psychological Reports, 65*, 818.

Lester, D. (1989b). Personal violence (suicide and homicide) in South Africa. *Acta Psychiatrica Scandinavica, 79*, 235-237.

Lester, D. (1994a). Differences in the epidemiology of suicide in Asian Americans by nation of origin. *Omega, 29*, 89-93.

Lester, D. (1994b). The epidemiology of suicide in Chinese population in six regions of the world. *Chinese Journal of Mental Health, 7*, 25-36.

Lester, D. (1994c). Suicide by jumping in Singapore as a function of high-rise apartment availability. *Perceptual and Motor Skills, 79*, 74.

Lester, D. (1994d). Suicide in immigrant groups as a function of their proportion in the country. *Perceptual and Motor Skills, 79*, 994.

Lester, D. (1996a, in press). Suicidal behavior in the enslaved in America. *Journal of Black Studies.*

Lester, D. (1996b). *Suicide in American Indians.* Commack, NY: Nova Science.

Lester, D., & Wilson, C. (1988). Suicide in Zimbabwe. *Central African Journal of Medicine, 34*, 147-149.

May, P. A., & Dizmang, L. H. (1974). Suicide and the American Indian. *Psychiatric Annals, 4*(11), 22-28.

Myers, L. J. (1993). *Understanding an Afrocentric world view.* Dubuque, IA: Kendall/Hunt.

Piersen, W. D. (1977). White cannibals, black martyrs. *Journal of Negro History, 62*, 147-159.

Sainsbury, P. (1973). Suicide. *Proceedings of the Royal Society of Medicine, 66*, 579-587.

Sainsbury, P., & Barraclough, B. M. (1968). Differences between suicide rates. *Nature, 220*, 1252.

Snelgrave, D. J. (1734). *A new account of some parts of Guinea and the slave trade.* London, J. & P. Knapton.

Sue, D. W., & Sue, D. (1990). *Counseling the culturally different.* New York: Wiley.

Van Winkle, N. W., & May, P. A. (1986). Native American suicide in New Mexico, 1959-1979. *Human Organization, 45*, 296-309.

Wallace, A. F. C. (1972). *The death and rebirth of the Seneca.* New York: Vintage.

Westermeyer, J. (1979). Ethnic identity problems among ten Indian psychiatric patients. *International Journal of Social Psychiatry, 25*, 188-197.

Zeisberger, D. (1910). David Zeisberger's history of the North American Indians. A. B. Hulbert & W. N. Schwarz (Eds.). *Ohio Archaeological and Historical Publications, 19*, 1-189.

7
Suicide: The Scourge of Native American People

Marlene EchoHawk, PHD

Reportedly, Native Americans have a rate of suicide that is greater than any other ethnic group in the United States, especially in the age range of 15–24. Many who are concerned as to why this is the case offer a variety of theories. Most of the theories have yet to be tested. This particular presentation focuses on the traditional tribal structure of most Native Americans and events of history that have impacted the cultures of Native American Tribes. The particular events covered refer to Western education, various religions, and legislation as playing a most significant role in impacting the cultures of Native Americans. With the hope that we can all work together to diminish the scourge of Native American people, I repeat the words of Chief Seattle, "... be just and deal kindly with my people."

Many Native American families throughout this country have experienced profound grief and pain due to the suicide of a family friend or relative. The number of suicide victims among Native American youth ages 15–24 is estimated to be three to four times higher than that of other ethnic groups. Although it is recognized that there is a need for immediate and ongoing professional counseling, there are serious questions regarding the availability of prevailing services that are able to respond in culturally sensitive and appropriate ways.

Although I appreciate the fact that I have acquired the academic training provided in the Western system, today I am going to share with you the knowledge I have acquired by growing up in a traditional Native American family. My hope is that I can give you good and useful information in order to promote a better spirit of cooperation between cultures.

My words, recorded here, concern the traditional tribal structure of most Native Americans, some of the historical factors that have impacted the cultures of Native Americans, how some tribes cope with death, the current status of many tribes, and finally the process of reclaiming our lives.

TRIBAL STRUCTURE

In order to conceptualize the way that traditional tribes existed and functioned as an organized group, it is helpful to use a circle. A circle is easy to visualize as well as commit to memory in connection with tribal structure.

Now visualize the circle as being divided into seven parts representing clans within the tribe. Some tribes have more than seven clans and some tribes have less, but I am using seven because that is the number of clans in my own tribe, the Otoe–Missouria Tribe of Oklahoma. The main point is that tribes are subdivided into clans or bands.

Marlene EchoHawk is Deputy Chief, Alcoholism and Substance Abuse Program Branch, Indian Health Service, Headquarters West, Albuquerque, NM 87110.

The author takes full responsibility for the contents of this paper. In no way does the author represent the views of the Indian Health Service or the Bureau of Indian Affairs. The author would like to express appreciation to Johanna Clevenger, MD, for authorizing participation in the American Association of Suicidology's annual conference.

The author respectfully dedicates this address to the memory of our Native American and Alaska Native youth who have blessed us here briefly before choosing to enter the spirit world.

Within each clan there is a further natural and recognized subdivision into biologically related families. However, all members within a clan or band are considered to be related irrespective of biological relationships. In essence, a clan constitutes members of the extended family.

The method of determining clan membership varies from tribe to tribe. The tribe used here determines clan membership on the father's side. This means that all children born within a marriage will automatically assume membership in the father's clan. Some tribes determine clanship on the mother's side, and still other tribes permit the mother and father to choose to which clan the child will belong, the mother's or father's clan, as each child is born.

Interdependence Supported by a Clan System

The strength in unity of purpose, philosophy, and belief system as seen through a logical analysis of the clan system helps us to understand the usefulness to social harmony that such an arrangement provided. It seems paradoxical to say that a tribe was divided to maintain cohesiveness but, in effect, that is the result of a subdivision into clans.

Each clan had an important function to perform for the survival and existence of the total group. For example, in the area of physical health, each clan had a "healer" or "healers" who might be skilled in one of the following areas: the control of hemorrhaging, setting and healing fractured bones, curing sick children, treating eye injuries and diseases, strokes and brain injuries, mental illnesses, and so forth. Not any one clan had "healers" in all of these areas, which meant that each clan was, more than likely, needed at some time by each of the other clans.

In the area of social development, certain relationships in the clan resulted in specific clan members assuming the role of teaching and maintaining social control.

Individual shaping of behavior occurred primarily within the biological family.

Moral development – the distinction between acceptable and unacceptable behaviors – was encouraged and taught through the recitation of legends and stories by grandparents to their grandchildren. This was a very important function of grandparents. For instance, if a child was disobedient, one of the grandparents might relate a story of a person who was disobedient and the bad consequences of such behavior. It would be left up to the child to identify or not identify with the character in the story. The stories would be appropriate to the age level of the child involved. Good behavior was also reinforced by verbal approval from the adults.

Briefly stated, the important responsibility assumed by each clan promoted the concept of interdependence. Members of each clan depended on members of every other clan, but all were depended on to make a contribution to the tribal group. This description of interdependence may clarify the stereotype of "noncompetitiveness" of Native American people. For one clan to compete with another clan would be viewed as extremely disrespectful and leading to dissension. Therefore, a sense of cooperation was encouraged throughout one's lifetime.

In summary, the clanship system provided the structure necessary for a tribe to maximize cooperation, which strengthened the tribal social system. Also, it is important to point out the advantage of this system to an individual's sense of identity from a psychological, emotional, and social viewpoint.

Clan and Biological Relationships

Specific roles and relationships existed within each clan. In addition to the usual biological relationships of parents, brothers, sisters, aunts, uncles, and grandparents, other relationships existed based on clan membership. To observe social protocol and to understand one's own role and responsibility within the family, clan, and tribe, it was vital to learn about relationships.

Members of a clan were considered to be related even though there were no biological relationships, and marriage within one's own clan was prohibited. In practice, the biological relationship generally took precedence over the clan relationship. The way two people can be related may overlap as a result of intermarriage.

One could be related to a person in such a way that talking to that person was prohibited. Silence, in some relationships, was considered a form of deep respect. Anyone who does not understand the nature of the relationships could easily misinterpret the silence as "poor family communication." Well-meaning efforts may be made to "help" the family communicate better. This may even be written up as a "goal" in a treatment plan. On the other hand, the family may actually need help in being able to communicate better. Therefore, it is extremely vital to have some understanding of tribal relationships to be able to differentiate social custom from actual pathology.

Role-Oriented Societies

Most tribes consider every person to be valuable, useful, and deserving of respect. As a way of emphasizing the importance of each individual, most tribes had various methods of integrating each newborn child into the clan and tribe.

In my own tribe, a child is considered to be a member of the father's clan. Later, the child was given a clan name, selected from among a variety of names "belonging" to the clan. The names were considered sacred and have existed for centuries within the same clan. No one was ever given the name of anyone who was still living.

The names were very meaningful for the individual as well as for the clan and tribe, and the child was encouraged to live up to the responsibility of his or her name. Young children learned to be proud of their names. A great deal of importance and ritual were associated with the naming ceremony. The names were timeless in their meaning and application. Bestowing of names was another practice through which Indian people gained a firm sense of identity and purpose.

Individuals brought up in this tradition were fortunate in establishing meaningful values that could always be applied within the context of their current lives.

Tribal cohesiveness achieved through the concept of close relationships, status, and roles (reinforced by ceremonializing of names) has undergone momentous changes. The chaos and social disarray that may be found today within Native American tribes and communities can be traced to the intervention of unfamiliar systems upon the tribes.

IMPACT OF SYSTEMS ON NATIVE AMERICAN TRIBES

Education

Native Americans have always been as concerned as all other cultures with the education of their children. However, the Native American method of teaching and the substance of what was considered important for children to learn differ from the typical Western educational system. It is not my intention to discuss how the two systems differ, but rather to point out how the Western system has impacted traditional tribal structure.

Mission Schools. The Western style of educating Native Americans began with the establishment of missionary schools by Roman Catholic groups in the mid-16th century (Berry, 1969). Mission schools were established primarily for the purpose of converting Native American people to Christianity. This missionary work was carried out mainly by the French Jesuits and Spanish Franciscans.

There was such a strong emphasis on the Christianizing of Native Americans that the academic area of the Jesuit mission schools was neglected. There seems to have been only enough secular education provided to ensure the conversion of the tribes to Christianity.

To say that mission schools were the "answer to the prayers" of Native Americans for their children would be inaccurate. Layman (1942) gives us some insight into the intervention of Native American parents with the school:

> Of the solicitude of the Indians for their children, Father Le Jeune wrote, "... these Barbarians cannot bear to have their children punished, nor even scolded, not being able to refuse anything to a crying child. They carry this to such an extent that upon the slightest pretext they would take them away from us, before they were educated." Thus the Jesuit priest stated one of the principal problems of Indian education, for throughout the entire history of the whiteman's attempts to educate the Indian, divergence in the attitudes of Indian parent and white teacher toward the treatment of children has been a source of conflict.

It is interesting to note that this conflict persists even up to the present time.

However, in order to do their work undisturbed, Native American children were taken from their families and required to live at the missions. Some Native American children were sent to France to learn the French language well enough to help the Jesuits in their mission schools.

The Catholic mission school efforts to Christianize Native Americans were followed by similar efforts by Protestant denominations. According to Berry (1969), "King James I, on March 24, 1617, called upon the Anglican clergy to collect money 'for the erecting of some churches and schools for ye education of ye children of these Barbarians in Virginia.'" Many Native Americans were taken to the College of William and Mary to be educated.

The Puritan influence of Reverend Eleazar Wheelock was felt by Native American tribes on the East Coast. The present Dartmouth College was originally founded by Reverend Wheelock for the purpose of Christianizing and teaching Native American children. His policy was to remove children from their families for the purpose of educating them. This group went one step farther by setting up an "outing system," which was an experiment "whereby Indian pupils were placed in Puritan homes during the vacation periods" (Berry, 1969).

Baptists, Presbyterians, Quakers, and Mormons, to name a few, have all engaged in efforts to educate Native American children.

Bureau of Indian Affairs Boarding Schools. The first off-reservation boarding school for Native Americans was established at Carlisle, Pennsylvania, in 1879; Army forts were converted into Indian schools following legislation in 1882; Indians were subsidized to attend public schools. In 1917 all government subsidies to religious groups for the purpose of educating Indian children were ended. This ushered in the era of the Bureau of Indian Affairs boarding schools (BIA schools).

Native American children were removed, sometimes forcibly, from their families to attend boarding schools long distances from their homes; the use of Indian languages by children was forbidden, with corporal punishment inflicted on those children found using their native languages. Students were sent out to live with White families during vacation times, and native religions were suppressed.

It was imagined that the Native American child, once enrolled in the school, would receive a basic education and emerge several years later as a "civilized" person. It was intended that the children reject the values and lifestyles of their parents. Although untrained teachers were the norm in rural American schools at that time (late 1800s), their employment in Indian schools often impeded the Indians' education, particularly when the teachers were not only untrained but also poorly educated. An Omaha Indian recalled the English the Native American children spoke

> was gathered from the imperfect comprehension of their books, the provincialism of the teachers, and the slang and bad grammar picked up from uneducated white persons employed at the school or at the Government Agent's. And because oddities of speech, profanity, localisms, and slang were unknown in the Omaha language, when such expres-

> sions fell upon the ears of these lads they innocently learned and used them without the slightest suspicion that there could be bad as well as good English. (LaFlesche, 1963)

Social Changes as a Result of a Non-Indian Education

The assimilation of Native American children into a society that was not their own has had a tremendous impact on tribal structure.

Every Native American child who became educated had to repudiate much of his or her own background—even though it was clear to the government that the benefits of White civilization were not, even when accessible, consistently preferred by the Native Americans.

The gulf created by the educators of Native American children has served to alter the cohesiveness of Native American tribes. Children educated in BIA schools were denied the affection of their parents. Parenting skills that would have been learned within their own families were lost. Their own native languages were soon forgotten, making communication with their own people difficult if not impossible.

Many "educated" Native American children in the late 1800s totally rejected the values and lifestyles of their parents.

Religion

If there were ever an area of "common ground" among Native American tribes, it can be said to have been in the area of a religious belief system. None of the tribes were without a belief in a supreme being. The outward manifestations of their various customs and traditions may have differed, but the general recognition of a "Great Spirit" did exist.

The first organized religious groups to influence Native American tribes away from their own traditional beliefs were those professing to be Christians. Among the earliest Christians to have contact with Native American people were missionary groups of the Roman Catholic church. The Jesuits were among the earliest missionary groups to work among Native American tribes, in the regions that we now refer to as the New England states and the Great Lakes area.

It will be conceded that the Christian zeal to win new converts to the practice of Christianity was the overriding motive behind the Jesuits' propensity to suffer great physical and mental hardships for their faith.

Many Protestant denominations have worked among Native American people to convert them to Christianity. It did not seem to matter whether the denomination was called Baptist, Episcopalian, Presbyterian, Quaker, or whatever, the aim and word of the missionary groups remained the same.

Berkhofer (1965) has pointed out that "Both missionaries and Indians recognized that the two cultural systems clashed, and the missionaries called the adherents of the two systems the Pagan Party and the Christian Party." We are given a very astute description by Berkhofer (1965) of the breakdown of tribal cohesiveness.

> Societal disruption naturally followed from missionarization, for the acceptance of new values as well as Pagan persecution demanded new social relationships. Sometimes conversion merely meant the end of polygamy. At other times couples separated because one spouse had been converted. In still other instances, people left their villages to settle in places more favorable to Indian Christianity. In extreme cases, new villages or bands were formed entirely of White-oriented Indians. Living, after the initial cultural divisions, the cleavage worsens, the community breaks into two physically separate groups which enables each one to live in its own community in which culture and social structure coincide. The process may repeat itself several times within the same original population.

Opposing views could only serve to fragment and disunite the tribes. A natural consequence of such disunity led to actual geographic relocation of opposing factions.

Legislation

Prior to the establishment of an American government, Native American tribes negotiated treaties with various colonial European groups settling on their lands. This practice recognized the sovereign status of tribes. Even after the American Revolution, when the United States Congress came into existence, treaties continued to be validated with Native American tribes on the basis of their being sovereign nations. Furthermore, the 1832 case of *Worcester v. Georgia* set the foundation of federal Indian law regarding territorial sovereignty for Indian tribes.

Colonial Years. The purpose of treaties negotiated before the original 13 colonies won their independence from Great Britain's domination was to gain access to Indian lands. The encroachment of European settlers had proceeded at such a rate that, in order to mollify the discontent of Indian tribes, the King of Britain issued the Proclamation of October 7, 1763. The purpose of the Proclamation was to prohibit the intrusion of settlers on land within the boundaries of Indian ownership and to regulate trade with Indians by unscrupulous European traders. Indians were placed under the protection of local officers directly responsible to the king.

The effect of avaricious large-scale engulfment of Indian lands resulted in the geographic dispersion of Indian tribes. At this point in history many tribes had already been fragmented by the impact of a non-Indian system of education and religion. Therefore, it became an easy matter for members of a tribe to physically move to a new location away from other members of the same tribe where there existed a difference in viewpoints.

The Issue of Sovereignty. As mentioned earlier, the case of *Worcester v. Georgia* established the tribes as territorial sovereigns. Furthermore, federal power over the regulation of Indian affairs took precedence over state power. The original judicial confirmation of Indian tribes as sovereign nations has since been modified by subsequent legislation. At the basis of conflicting legislation is the issue of sovereignty.

The recognition of tribal sovereignty is considered to be just and humane. Nevertheless, the notion of territorial sovereignty loses some of its potency when it must be acknowledged that large land grabs, referred to earlier, diminished the territory over which a tribe could be sovereign. While the support of tribal sovereignty itself did not fragment the tribe—actually just the contrary—the controversy surrounding independent Indian nations served to sabotage efforts of Indian tribes to achieve their former autonomous status.

The most serious legislative effort to "assimilate" Indians occurred with the passage of the General Allotment Act in 1887. Other names for this act are the Dawes Act or Dawes Severalty Act. The primary purpose of this legislation was to open more land for non-Indian settlement, but ostensibly it was intended to "release" Indians from government wardship. In effect, tribal lands were broken up for individual distribution to tribal members. Individual allottees were prohibited from selling or mortgaging their parcel of land for a period of 25 years. Wholesale Indian land sales took place at the end of that 25-year period.

I have just briefly touched on major historical legislative decisions that have played a role in the process of disrupting tribal cohesiveness. A detailed presentation of all treaties negotiated and other legislative decisions, however important, is not possible nor appropriate within the context of this address.

From 1778 to 1871, the United States Senate ratified 371 treaties with Indian tribes. On March 3, 1871, Congress passed a bill prohibiting further treaty making with tribes. This bill did not invalidate treaties that had been negotiated up to that point.

As a result of the broad systematic

changes described, tribal unity was disrupted, to some extent, among all Indian tribes. A Western education, missionaries, and legislative acts may be considered to have exerted the greatest influence on weakening and fragmenting tribal unity by erecting language barriers, undermining parental influence, introducing nontraditional religions, uprooting tribes from their lands, so on, and so on.

Other events were taking place as well. Examples of these are intertribal and interracial marriages, a change in the methods of rearing children, widespread alcohol usage among the tribes, the quality and quantity of food consumed. All served to influence the social framework of daily life for Indian people.

CURRENT STATUS OF NATIVE AMERICANS

Although it is not possible to quantify the many changes that have occurred across and within the tribes, one thing is certain—major changes have taken place among the tribes that have survived.

It is estimated that at least 10 million Native Americans once lived and flourished throughout what is now the United States. The 1990 census identified over 2 million people of Native American or Alaska Native heritage. The majority of the Native American population are members of the more than 545 federally recognized Native American tribes, bands, pueblos, and villages.

Many social and economic problems exist in Native American communities, not the least of which is suicide. The profound grief related to the loss of a loved one is made somewhat easier because the entire community comes together to mourn the loss and support the survivors.

To emphasize the Native American peoples' view of an afterlife, I would like to use the words of the great orator Chief Seattle in 1853 when Governor Isaac Stevens asked to buy his tribe's land:

> Our departed braves, fond mothers, glad happy-hearted maidens, and even our little children who lived here and rejoiced here for a brief season, will love these somber solitudes, and at eventide they greet shadowy returning spirits. And when the last red man shall have perished, and the memory of my tribe shall have become a myth among the white men, these shores will swarm with the invisible dead of my tribe, and when your children's children think themselves alone in the field, the store, the shop, upon the highway or in the silence of the woods, they will not be alone. In all the earth there is no place dedicated to solitude. At night, when the streets of your cities and villages shall be silent, and you think them deserted, they will throng with the returning hosts that once filled and still love this beautiful land. The white man will never be alone. Let him be just and deal kindly with my people. For the dead are not powerless. Dead, did I say? There is no death. Only a change of worlds. (Nerburn, 1994)

RECLAIMING OUR LIVES

Native American Tribes and Alaska Natives now have the opportunity to run many of their own programs that are currently managed by the Indian Health Service as well as the Bureau of Indian Affairs. Many tribes have already exercised their option to maintain their own programs that they consider more relevant to their cultural needs. However, some tribes still prefer to let the two agencies manage the services related to health and educational needs. The self-determination efforts have yet to be evaluated, but the cultural aspect of services can be implemented based on the tribe's wishes.

Many Native Americans may still come to the attention of our mental health clinics who do not live near services for which they may qualify. It is for this reason that I presented the information regarding the cultural breakdown and other gross injustices perpetrated upon indigenous people. Questionable practices are still around up to the present time. Indigenous clients must be allowed to grieve and talk about their feelings of historical trauma, alienation, and poor sense of identity. Acceptance of their spiritual practices must be encouraged and viewed as high priority. Sensitive people need few reminders.

With the hope that we can all work together to diminish the scourge of Native

American people, I repeat the words of Chief Seattle, "... be just and deal kindly with my people."

REFERENCES

Berkhofer, R. (1960). *Protestant missionaries to the American Indian, 1787–1862.* Doctoral dissertation, Cornell University.

Berry, B. (1969). *The education of American Indians: A survey of the literature.* Washington, DC: U.S. Government Printing Office. (Document No. 24-230)

LaFlesche, F. (1963). *The middle five: Indian schoolboys of the Omaha Tribe.* Madison: University of Wisconsin Press.

Layman, M. (1942). *A history of Indian education in the United States.* Doctoral dissertation, University of Minnesota.

Nerburn, K. (1994). *The wisdom of the Great Chiefs, The classic speeches of Chief Red Jacket, Chief Joseph and Chief Seattle, The classic wisdom collection.* San Rafal, CA: New World Library.

8
African-American Suicide: A Cultural Paradox

Jewelle Taylor Gibbs, MSW, PhD

African-American suicide rates have traditionally been lower than White rates despite a legacy of racial discrimination, persistent poverty, social isolation, and lack of community resources. This paper focuses on four issues: (1) patterns and trends of Black suicide across the lifespan; (2) risk and protective factors in subgroups of Blacks; (3) the influence of cultural factors on suicide patterns of Blacks; and (4) implications of these patterns for prevention and early intervention of suicidal behavior among African Americans. Risk factors for Black suicide include: male sex, early adulthood, substance abuse, psychiatric disorders, family or interpersonal conflict, antisocial behavior, and homosexuality. Protective factors that mitigate the risks of suicide include religiosity, older age, southern residence, and social support. Implications for preventive policies and programs are discussed to counter the recent trend of rising suicide rates among adolescents and very elderly Blacks.

Throughout a turbulent history of slavery, legal segregation, civil rights protests, and controversy over affirmative action, African Americans have traditionally had low suicide rates compared to White Americans (Griffith & Bell, 1989; Heckler, 1985). Despite generations of racial discrimination, persistent poverty, social and cultural isolation, and lack of community resources, suicide rates among Blacks have also remained relatively low compared to other ethnic minority groups in American society (Earls, Escobar, & Manson, 1990). This phenomenon has puzzled many social scientists because of the apparent paradox between the disadvantaged status of African Americans and their infrequent use of suicide as a solution to their problems.

Patterns of suicide among African Americans are dissimilar in many respects from those of Anglo-Americans, although some similar trends between these two groups have recently emerged. Research on African-American suicide has identified distinctive patterns of suicidal behavior among Black adults (Bush, 1976; Davis, 1979; Swanson & Breed, 1976); Black adolescents and youth (Baker, 1990; Gibbs, 1988; Rutledge, 1990); Black women (Alston & Anderson, 1995; Howze, 1977); and the Black elderly (Baker, 1994; Seiden, 1982). Further, some researchers have identified sex differences in patterns of suicide of Black males and females (Bingham, Bennion, Openshaw, & Adams, 1994; Gibbs & Hines, 1989; Kirk & Zucker, 1979). Few studies have compared suicidal behavior between Black and other non-White groups (Frederick, 1984; Heacock, 1990; Wyche & Rotheram-Borus, 1990).

Official suicide statistics are plagued with methodological problems that seriously affect their validity and reliability (Monk, 1987; Shaffer & Fisher, 1981; Warshauer & Monk, 1978). As researchers have noted, Black suicide statistics are questionable due to such factors as misreporting of accidental or undetermined deaths, state and regional variations in reporting, and cultural attitudes of family members who feel stigmatized by a relative's suicide (Gibbs, 1988a; Peck, 1983).

In their analysis of suicide data, Phil-

Jewelle Taylor Gibbs is a professor in the School of Social Welfare at the University of California at Berkeley, Berkeley, CA 94720.

Suicide and Life-Threatening Behavior, Vol. 27(1), Spring 1997

lips and Ruth (1993) concluded that rates for African Americans and females are most likely to be underreported in official statistics, thus raising concerns about using these data for research and public policy.

This paper has two goals: to identify some of the cultural factors associated with low suicide rates among African Americans, and to propose some socioeconomic and political factors that are contributing to rising rates of suicide among Black youth and the elderly. The paper focuses on four major issues: (1) current patterns and rates of suicide across the life span; (2) risk and protective factors in subgroups of Blacks; (3) cultural factors influencing suicide patterns in the Black community; and (4) implications of these patterns for prevention and early intervention of suicide and suicidal behavior among African Americans.

RATES AND PATTERNS OF AFRICAN-AMERICAN SUICIDE

African-American suicide rates show a different developmental trajectory over the life span than rates for Anglo-Americans or other non-White groups. In general, suicide rates for Blacks are very low in adolescence, increase in young adulthood, then decrease with age, reaching a peak between the ages of 25 and 34. Compared to Blacks, rates for Whites are relatively high in adolescence and young adulthood, then increase with age, reaching a peak between the ages of 75 and 84 (see Table 1) (National Center for Health Statistics, 1994).

African-American Youth

For all youth between 15 and 24, the suicide rate doubled between 1960 and 1989 but leveled off between 1979 and 1984 (Bingham et al., 1994). However, between 1986 and 1991, while the rate remained stable for females (15–19) in all ethnic groups, the suicide rate among Black males was increasing at a faster rate than among White males (Shaffer, Gould, & Hicks, 1994). Thus, although Black males and females, 15–19, still have lower rates overall than White males and females, there has been a sudden and sharp recent increase among young Black males that warrants attention (see Table 2).

In their analysis of youth suicide rates, Bingham and his colleagues (1994) showed that the rates in all ethnic groups increased rapidly across the age levels from 10–14, 15–19, and 20–24. Although this study found that Blacks at all three age levels had substantially lower suicide rates than Whites and "other" non-Whites, Black females were found to have the lowest rate of suicide of all sex–race–age groups.

Ethnic and gender differences were also found, with White youth significantly more likely than Blacks to commit suicide by ingesting gas, hanging, or using "other firearms." Females preferred drugs as their first choice of method, but Black females still had the lowest suicide rates in this category (Bingham et al., 1994).

African-American Adults

From 1980 to 1992, overall rates of suicide increased for Black males from 11.1 to 12.3 per 100,000, while simultaneously decreasing for Black females from 2.4 to 2.0 per 100,000 (Centers for Disease Control and Prevention, 1995). During this period, Black male suicide rates exhibited an upward trend in three major age groups: 15–24, 45–54, and 75–84, leveling off by 1992. For males, ages 35–44, the suicide rate was fairly stable but increased slightly in 1992. Among Black male adults, those in the 25–34 age group consistently showed the highest suicide rates (see Table 1).

By contrast, among Black females, the suicide rates showed a slight downward trend in all age groups except those in the 65- to 74-year-old age group. Since 1980, women in the 25–34 and 35–44 age groups have been slightly more likely to commit suicide than those in the 45–54 age group, although these differences are minor (see Table 1). Black males are four to six times

TABLE 1
Suicide Rates per 100,000 According to Sex, Race, and Age: 1960-1992

Age (years)	1960	1970	1980	1985	1992
Male					
White					
15–24	8.6	13.9	21.4	22.7	22.5
25–34	14.9	19.9	25.6	25.4	24.7
35–44	21.9	23.3	23.5	23.5	25.2
45–54	33.7	29.5	24.2	25.1	24.0
55–64	40.2	35.0	25.8	28.6	26.0
65–74	42.0	38.7	32.5	35.3	32.0
75–84	55.7	45.5	45.5	57.1	53.0
85–	61.3	50.3	52.8	60.3	67.6
Black					
15–24	4.1	10.5	12.3	13.3	17.3
25–34	12.4	19.2	21.8	19.6	19.2
35–44	12.8	12.6	15.6	14.9	16.9
45–54	10.8	13.8	12.0	13.5	12.4
55–64	16.2	10.6	11.7	11.5	10.1
65–74	11.3	8.7	11.1	15.8	11.8
75–84	6.6	8.9	10.5	15.6	18.5
85–	6.9	10.3	18.8	7.7	17.1
Female					
White					
15–24	2.3	4.2	4.6	4.7	4.1
25–34	5.8	9.0	7.5	6.4	5.0
35–44	8.1	13.0	9.1	7.7	7.2
45–54	10.9	13.5	10.2	9.0	7.9
55–64	10.9	12.3	9.1	8.4	7.2
65–74	8.8	9.6	7.0	7.3	6.3
75–84	9.2	7.2	5.7	7.0	6.6
85–	6.1	6.1	5.8	4.7	6.3
Black					
15–24	1.3	3.8	2.3	2.0	2.1
25–34	3.0	5.7	4.1	3.0	4.3
35–44	3.0	3.7	4.6	3.6	3.3
45–54	3.1	3.7	2.8	3.2	3.0
55–64	3.0	2.0	2.3	2.2	2.0
65–74	2.3	2.9	1.7	2.0	2.0
75–84	1.3	1.7	1.4	4.5	–
85–	–	3.2	–	1.4	3.0

Sources: National Center for Health Statistics, *Vital Statistics of the United States, 1991*, Vol. 2, *Mortality, Part A* (Hyattsville, MD: Public Health Service, 1994) and Centers for Disease Control, *Suicide in the United States, 1980-1992* (Atlanta, GA: National Center for Injury Prevention and Control, 1995).

more likely to commit suicide and to use more lethal means than Black females. They are also more likely to take their own lives in young adulthood (25–34), although the highest risk period for Black females has shifted from middle adulthood (35–44) to young adulthood since 1985 (see Table 1).

Overall rates of suicide among White males increased from 18.8 to 19.4 per 100,000 from 1980 to 1992 (Centers for Disease Control and Prevention, 1995).

TABLE 2
Suicide Rates per 100,000 by Sex, Race, and Age Group: 1980–1991

Age (years)	Total			Male White			Male Black			Female White			Female Black		
	1980	1990	1991	1980	1990	1991	1980	1990	1991	1980	1990	1991	1980	1990	1991
All ages	11.9	12.4	12.2	19.9	22.0	21.7	10.3	12.0	12.1	5.9	5.3	5.2	2.2	2.3	1.9
10 to 14	0.8	1.5	1.5	1.4	2.3	2.4	0.5	1.6	2.0	0.3	0.9	0.8	0.1	–	–
15 to 19	8.5	11.1	11.0	15.0	19.3	19.1	5.6	11.5	12.2	3.3	4.0	4.2	1.6	1.9	–
20 to 24	16.1	15.1	14.9	27.8	26.8	26.5	20.0	19.0	20.7	5.9	4.4	4.3	3.1	2.6	1.8
25 to 34	16.0	15.2	15.2	25.6	25.6	26.1	21.8	21.9	21.1	7.5	6.0	5.8	4.1	3.7	3.3
35 to 44	15.4	15.3	14.7	23.5	25.3	24.7	15.6	16.9	15.2	9.1	7.4	7.2	4.6	4.0	2.9

Source: U.S. National Center for Health Statistics, Monthly Vital Statistics Report and unpublished data, *Statistical Abstract of the United States* (Washington, DC: U.S. Government Printing Office, 1994).

White male suicide rates remained fairly stable across age groups, except for major increases in the 75–84 and over-85 age groups, which leveled off in 1992 (see Table 1). For White males, the highest risk periods are for men in the 65 years and older age groups, following retirement; whereas Black males in early adulthood are most at risk for suicide. Since 1980 White male suicide rates have averaged about 60% higher than the rate for Black males.

The overall suicide rate for White females also decreased between 1980 and 1992 from 5.7 to 4.6 per 100,000 (Centers for Disease Control and Prevention, 1995). In contrast to Black women, the highest rates of suicide among White women is in the 45–54 age group, but they also have higher rates than Blacks among all women over age 65 (see Table 1). White female suicide rates have also consistently been more than twice as high as rates for Black females since 1970 (see Table 1).

African-American Elderly

Black elderly suicide rates have been significantly lower than rates of elderly Whites, particularly among older females. However, since 1970 the rates have increased dramatically among Black males, 65 years and older (Blazer, 1991; Meehan, Saltzman, & Sattin, 1991). In the over-85 age group, the rate has risen between 1970 and 1992 from 10.3 to 17.1 per 100,000, with wide fluctuations in the 22-year period (see Table 1). For older Black females, the suicide rate has been more stable, punctuated by moderate increases with no predictable pattern. The disparity between the rates for Black males and Black females increases with age, further exacerbating the preexisting imbalances in the male–female ratios and available marriage partners in the Black community.

Since 1970 suicide rates for very elderly Black and White males have followed an upward trend. However, in the 75–84 age group, the White male suicide rate has generally shown a slower rate of growth than the rate for Black males and has actually declined since 1985. But in the over-85 age group, the White male suicide rate has increased sharply from 50.3 to 67.6 per 100,000 in 1992, whereas the trend for Black males has fluctuated with no consistent pattern from 10.3 to 17.1 per 100,000 (see Table 1).

Suicide rates for Black and White elderly females have also fluctuated since 1970 (National Center for Health Statistics, 1994). Between 1970 and 1992, suicide rates of Black females over age 65 decreased or remained fairly stable in each subgroup except in the over-85 age group, which registered an increase in 1992 (see Table 1). Similarly, the suicide rate for White females over age 65 also declined from their 1970 levels, except in the over-85 age group, where the 1992 rate was slightly higher than the 1970 rate (6.3 vs. 6.1 per 100,000).

Since 1970, in general, suicide rates for White females over 65 years of age have been two to four times higher than those for Black females. The disparity between the rates of Black and White females appears to be greatest in the 65- to 74-year age group, the period when retirement usually occurs and women are frequently widowed. Since older Black women tend to have higher rates of poverty and chronic illnesses than their White counterparts, their lower suicide rate at this stage is counterintuitive and suggests some protective factors or coping skills that mitigate against suicidal behavior.

RISK AND PROTECTIVE FACTORS IN AFRICAN-AMERICAN SUICIDE

A review of recent literature on suicidal behavior in African Americans provides a multidisciplinary perspective on risk and protective factors and other variables associated with this self-destructive behavior.

Risk Factors in African-American Suicide

Researchers have identified the following risk factors for suicide among Blacks:

1. Male sex – Black males are four to six times more likely to commit suicide than Black females (Baker, 1990; Gibbs & Hines, 1989).
2. Age – young adult Blacks between the ages of 25 and 34 (for males and females) are more likely to commit suicide than either younger or older age groups (Frierson & Lippmann, 1990; Maris, 1995).
3. Substance abuse – high rates of suicide and suicide attempts are associated with abuse of alcohol or drugs, for both youth and adults (Earle, Forquer, Volo, & McDonnell, 1994; Frierson & Lippmann, 1990; Murphy, Wetzel, Robins, & McEvoy, 1992).
4. Depression – high rates of suicide and suicidal behavior are found among youth and adults who are depressed (Adcock, Nagy, & Simpson, 1991; Kirk & Zucker, 1979; Rotheram-Borus, 1993).
5. Family dysfunction, conflict, or violence – high rates of suicide are found among adolescents who experience family conflict, abuse, or violence (Howze, 1977; Summerville, Kaslow, Abbata, & Cronan, 1994; Topol & Resnikoff, 1982).
6. Interpersonal discord/marital conflict – youth and women who experience intense interpersonal conflict also have high rates of suicide (Baker, 1990; Hendin, 1978; Wilson, 1981).
7. Acting out/delinquency – youth with a history of acting out or delinquency are at higher risk for suicide or suicidal behavior (Gibbs, 1982; Kempton & Forehand, 1992; Neigher & Hopkins, 1988).
8. Psychiatric disorders/psychological symptomatology – high rates of psychiatric disorders or symptomatology are reported among youth and adults who engage in suicidal behavior (Frierson & Lippmann, 1990; Summerville, et al., 1992; Trautman, Rotheram-Borus, Dopkins, & Lewin, 1991).
9. Homosexuality/AIDS – higher rates of suicide are found among young Black homosexual males and those infected with HIV or AIDS (Proctor & Groze, 1994; Ramafedi, Farrow, & Deisher, 1991; Rotheram-Borus, Hunter, & Rosario, 1994).

In a regional analysis of African-American suicides, Lester (1990-91) found that rates were higher in the North and in states with higher rates of unemployment. In a related study, Lester (1990-91) found an association between higher Black suicide rates and higher education, higher income, and lower fertility rates, correlates that seem to contradict conventional beliefs about suicide in minority populations.

In summary, the combination of male gender, early adulthood, and substance abuse may be associated with heightened vulnerability and an increased suicide risk for Blacks.

Protective Factors in African-American Suicide

Researchers have identified the following protective factors that reduce suicide risk among Blacks:

1. Religiosity – church attendance or affiliation is associated with lower rates of suicide (Early, 1992; Martin, 1984).
2. Old age – suicide rates tend to decline with age among Blacks, although there has been a recent increase in suicide among very elderly Blacks (Blazer, 1991; Meehan, Saltzman, & Sattin, 1991).
3. Southern region – Black suicide rates tend to be lower in the south and in areas with less racial integration (Hickman, 1984; Lester, 1990-91; Shaffer, Gould, & Hicks, 1994).
4. Social support – Black suicide rates tend to be higher among those who live alone and are not involved in family units (Davis, 1980; Dunston, 1990; Gibbs & Martin, 1964).

To summarize, the combination of strong religious beliefs, social support, and ethnic neighborhoods may mitigate against the effects of aging and poverty for Blacks, thus reducing their suicide risk.

Other Factors Associated with Suicide in African Americans

Several researchers have found that White youth and adults more frequently report suicidal ideations than Blacks as a possible precursor to suicidal behavior (Lester & Anderson, 1992; Molock et al., 1994). Similarly, self-reported depression is more frequently associated with suicidal attempts in White than in Black youth (Kempton & Forehand, 1992; Summerville et al., 1992).

These findings suggest that clinicians should be cautious about using self-reports of depression and suicidal ideations as predictors of suicidal behaviors in Black youth, who might act out as a defense against feelings of sadness (Gibbs, 1988a).

Black males, responding to feelings of anger and alienation, sometimes engage in violent confrontations with the police, family, or peers, resulting in victim-precipitated homicide, arguably a form of extreme suicidal behavior (Gibbs, 1988a).

Finally, the easy availability of guns in the inner city is a significant factor in the rising rates of suicide and homicide of Black youth and adults, many of whom are chronically frustrated and often impulsively direct their aggression against themselves as well as against others (Bingham et al., 1994; Frierson & Lippmann, 1990; Gibbs, 1992).

INFLUENCE OF CULTURAL PATTERNS ON AFRICAN-AMERICAN SUICIDE RATES

African-American cultural values underlying the protective factors that reduce suicidal risk can be delineated in five domains: (1) the role of religion, (2) the role of the Black woman, (3) the role of the elder, (4) the role of the extended family, and (5) the role of a cohesive social environment (cf. Early, 1992; Gibbs, 1988a).

First, religiosity is perhaps the most important protective factor for Blacks, the majority of whom are affiliated with Protestant denominations such as Baptists and Methodists, which represent a strong fundamentalist tradition that condemns suicide as sinful (Early, 1992). The Black church has also traditionally served as a source of social cohesion, social support, and stress reduction for the African-American community (Billingsley, 1992; Lincoln & Mamiya, 1990).

Religious beliefs have undoubtedly influenced the cultural beliefs of many African Americans that "suicide is a white thing," as Early (1992) characterized it. Since the days of slavery, one of the major functions of religion has been to provide a philosophical rationale for Blacks to endure poverty and discrimination in this life for the promise of a better life in the hereafter. Thus African Americans have subscribed to the values of endurance, resilience, and persistence in the face of adversity (Billingsley, 1992; Hill, 1972). From this perspective of fortitude in dealing with life's challenges, suicide has been viewed as an unacceptable solution, a sign of submission, and a certain route to eternal damnation (Branch, 1988).

In addition to their life-affirming philosophy, Black church leaders have played a major role in the Civil Rights Movement, providing their members with a sense of purpose and a spirit of group solidarity, and promoting a collective sense of empowerment and positive group identity (Billingsley, 1992; Branch, 1988).

Second, the central role of women in the Black community may be a significant factor in their low suicide rates. The courage and resilience of Black women in surviving slavery, nurturing their families, and building their communities has been well documented (Giddings, 1984; Stack 1974). Black women have learned to cope with high levels of stress, poverty, and discrimination by forming strong social networks, sharing resources, assuming flexible family roles, and turning to religion as a source of comfort for their feelings of anger and depression (Gibbs & Fuery, 1994; Greene, 1994; Myers, 1980). These strategies have enabled Black women to develop effective ways to ward off depression and to counter the risk of suicide. However, intense and chronic feelings of anger, frustration, or hopelessness may precipitate nonfatal suicidal behavior in some Black women (Alston &

Anderson, 1995; Hendin, 1969; Howze, 1977).

Third, elders play an important role in the African-American community and are treated with respect and dignity as mentors. In contrast to the Anglo-American elderly, a higher proportion of Black elders live independently or in their extended families rather than in nursing homes or retirement communities (Beck & Beck, 1989). Moreover, many Blacks look forward to retirement from low-status, low-wage jobs. Black elders continue to function after retirement in important roles as heads of households, caretakers of children, part-time workers, and volunteers (Jackson, 1980; Minkler & Roe, 1993). This transition is particularly true of Black women, who typically live longer than their spouses and male peers, a situation that may account for the negligible rates of suicide in Black women over 75 years of age.

Fourth, the extended family and kin networks have played a major role in the survival of African Americans in a frequently hostile society, fulfilling a number of important functions such as economic support, emotional support, and social support (cf. Billingsley, 1992; Hill, 1972; McAdoo, 1981). In the absence of social agencies to provide essential services for disadvantaged Blacks in the South, the extended family, kin networks, and the African-American church filled those needs, ranging from rearing orphaned children to caring for the chronically ill and the infirm elderly (cf. Billingsley, 1992; Greene, 1994; Lincoln, 1990).

Thus, the extended family served as a buffer between its members and the stresses of the external environment, providing them with a sense of identity, security, and support, and reducing the risk of suicide among rural and low-income Blacks. In recent years, this family form has diminished among Blacks as they have migrated from the rural South to the urban North and West, and have generally become more affluent, leaving the inner-city disadvantaged families behind in deteriorating communities (Wilson, 1987).

Fifth, the cohesive social environment of ethnic neighborhoods has reinforced the role of the extended family. Findings that Black suicide rates are lower in the South and higher in areas with smaller proportions of Blacks in the population suggest that, in communities where Blacks are less integrated, they might experience greater social cohesion, particularly in cities where the Black community is geographically and socially segregated (Lester, 1990–91; Shaffer, Gould & Hicks, 1994). Ironically, Blacks in segregated communities may experience less status anxiety and social rejection than in the integrated communities where their social status is less clear and their interracial interactions more ambivalent (Gibbs & Martin, 1964).

For example, the rate of increase in youth suicide has been greatest among Black youth in the North and West, areas with relatively low Black populations. As Shaffer and his colleagues (1994, p. 1811) suggest, this increase may reflect "an accelerating pace of occupational, residential, political, and educational integration" that, in turn, leads to a process of "deculturation" and subsequently results in higher rates of suicide among those Blacks who are cut off from the social cohesion and cultural identity of the Black community.

In fact, the social and psychological benefits of a cohesive Black community have been considerably weakened by massive changes such as integration, urbanization, deindustrialization, and secularization of the broader society. Ironically, these "progressive" changes may have contributed to a declining sense of community and fewer social supports for vulnerable Blacks.

SUMMARY AND CONCLUSIONS

This paper reviews the patterns of African-American suicide across the life span, the risk and protective factors, and notes the relationship between suicide rates and indices of racial integration and social mobility.

During the decades of the 1960s and 1970s Black youth were heavily involved in social action through civil rights and antiwar protests, both of which offered them a sense of meaning and expectations of increased educational and economic opportunity. By the end of the 1980s, Black youth had seen limits imposed on their aspirations, dwindling opportunities, and a government retreat from affirmative action (Orfield & Ashkinaze, 1991).

The rise in suicide rates from 1986 to 1991 for young Black males may very well reflect their feelings of disappointment and despair over these dwindling opportunities. These higher rates might also be partly attributed to the increasing levels of unemployment, gangs, drugs, and violence in the inner cities (cf. Gibbs, 1988b; Taylor, 1995). Since acting out and substance abuse are both associated with increased suicide risk, some of these young men may commit suicide as the ultimate act of self-destruction, a way out of their chronic feelings of anger and frustration. In our recent study of Black youth in south central Los Angeles, we found a pervasive sense of hopelessness and despair among youth who were school dropouts and chronically unemployed (Gibbs & Bankhead-Greene, 1996).

IMPLICATIONS FOR PREVENTION AND EARLY INTERVENTION

Prevention strategies to reverse this trend of higher Black youth suicide rates should focus on increasing life options for these youth by increasing high school graduation rates, strengthening job training programs, and increasing employment opportunities in semiskilled, skilled, and technical occupations (Gibbs, 1988; Orfield & Ashkinaze, 1991).

Additionally, school-based health clinics should be established in inner-city high schools and junior high schools, where a range of services could be offered to address mental and physical health problems such as depression, posttraumatic stress symptoms, grief reactions, substance abuse, teen pregnancy, and a host of other conditions that impact negatively on an adolescent's self-esteem and feelings of competence (Gibbs, 1990).

Early intervention strategies should focus on identifying those youth at risk for suicidal behavior because of specific social, personal, and behavioral characteristics, such as those from dysfunctional and abusive families, gay and lesbian youth, and youth with histories of psychological problems or self-destructive behaviors (substance abuse, delinquency, suicidal attempts). These at-risk youth could particularly benefit from crisis intervention, peer counseling, or youth development programs that include mentoring and career counseling.

Programs that improve economic self-sufficiency and enhance family functioning are needed to provide incentives to young adults who need employment and support to raise families, while elderly Blacks are most concerned about social insurance and health benefits to maintain their independence and dignity.

Without concerted efforts to develop a comprehensive set of public policies to address these developmental, social, and economic needs of Black and other low-income minority groups, African-American suicide rates will probably continue to rise as the risk factors will inevitably outweigh the protective factors that have kept these rates surprisingly low for generations.

REFERENCES

Adcock, A. G., Nagy, S., & Simpson, J. A. (1991). Selected risk factors in adolescents with suicide attempts. *Adolescence, 26*(104), 817–828.

Albers, E., & Evans, W. (1994). Suicide ideation among a stratified sample of rural and urban adolescents. *Child and Adolescent Social Work Journal, 11*(5), 379–389.

Allen, W. R. (1978). Black family research in the United States: A review, assessment and extension. *Journal of Comparative Family Studies, 9,* 168–189.

Alston, M., & Anderson, S. (1995). Suicidal behavior in African-American women. In S. Canetto & D.

Lester (Eds.), *Women and suicidal behavior* (pp. 133-143). New York: Springer.

Baker, F. M. (1990). Black youth suicide: Literature review with a focus on prevention. *Journal of the National Medical Association, 82*(7), 495-507.

Baker, F. M. (1994). Suicide among ethnic minority elderly: A statistical and psychosocial perspective. *Journal of Geriatric Psychiatry, 27*(2), 241-264.

Beck, R. W., & Beck, S. H. (1989). The incidence of extended households among middle-aged black and white women. *Journal of Family Issues, 10*, 147-168.

Belle, D. (1982). *Lives in stress: Women and depression.* Beverly Hills, CA: Sage.

Billingsley, A. (1992). *Climbing Jacob's ladder: The enduring legacy of African-American families.* New York: Simon & Schuster.

Bingham, C. R., Bennion, L. D., Openshaw, D. K., & Adams, G. R. (1994). An analysis of age, gender and racial differences in recent national trends of youth suicide. *Journal of Adolescence, 17*, 53-71.

Blazer, D. G. (1991). Suicide risk factors in the elderly: An epidemiological study. *Journal of Geriatric Psychiatry, 24*(2), 175-190.

Branch, T. (1988). *Parting the Waters: America in the King years.* New York: Simon and Schuster.

Bush, J. (1976). Suicide and Blacks: A conceptual framework. *Suicide and Life-Threatening Behavior, 6*(4), 216-222.

Canetto, S. S., & Lester, D. (Eds.) (1995). *Women and suicidal behavior.* New York: Springer.

Centers for Disease Control and Prevention. (1995). *Suicide in the United States: 1980-1992.* Atlanta, GA: National Center for Injury Prevention and Control.

Davis, R. (1979). Black suicide in the seventies: Current trends. *Suicide and Life-Threatening Behavior, 8*(3), 161-173.

Davis, R. (1980). Suicide among young blacks: Trends and perspectives. *Phylon, 41*(3), 223-229.

Dressler, W. (1985). Extended family relationships, social support, and mental health in a Southern Black community. *Journal of Health and Social Behavior, 26*, 39-48.

Dunston, P. J. (1990). Stress, coping, and social support: Their effects on black women. In D. S. Ruiz (Ed.), *Handbook of mental health and mental disorders among Black Americans* (pp. 133-147). New York: Greenwood Press.

Earle, K. A., Forquer, S. L., Volo, A. M., & McDonnell, P. M. (1994). Characteristics of outpatient suicides. *Hospital and Community Psychiatry, 45*(2), 123-126.

Earls, F., Escobar, J., & Manson, S. M. (1990). Suicide in minority groups: Epidemiologic and cultural perspectives. In S. J. Blumenthal & D. J. Kupfer (Eds.), *Suicide over the life cycle: Risk factors, assessment and treatment of suicidal patients* (pp. 571-598). Washington, DC: American Psychiatric Press.

Early, K. E. (1992). *Religion and suicide in the African-American community.* Westport, CT: Greenwood Press.

Edelman, M. W. (1987). *Families in peril: An agenda for social change.* Cambridge, MA: Harvard University Press.

Frederick, C. J. (1984). Suicide in young minority group persons. In H. Sudak, A. Ford, & N. Rushforth (Eds.), *Suicide in the young.* Boston, MA: John Wright.

Frierson, R. L., & Lippmann, S. B. (1990). Attempted suicide by black men and women: An 11 year study. *Journal of the Kentucky Medical Association, 88*(6), 287-292.

Garrison, C. Z., Addy, C. L., Jackson, K. L., McKeown, R. E., et al. (1991). A longitudinal study of suicidal ideation in young adolescents. *Journal of the American Academy of Child and Adolescent Psychiatry, 30*(4), 597-603.

Gibbs, J. T. (1982). Depression and suicidal behavior among delinquent females: Ethnic and sociocultural variations. *Journal of Clinical Psychology, 38*, 159-167.

Gibbs, J. T. (1988a). Conceptual, methodological, and sociocultural issues in Black youth suicide: Implications for assessment and early intervention. *Suicide and Life-Threatening Behavior, 18*, 73-89.

Gibbs, J. T. (Ed.) (1988b). *Young, Black and male in America: An endangered species.* Westport, CT: Greenwood Press.

Gibbs, J. T. (1990). Mental health issues of Black adolescents: Implications for policy and practice. In A. R. Stiffman & L. E. Davis (Eds.), *Ethnic issues in adolescent mental health* (pp. 21-52). Newbury Park, CA: Sage Publications.

Gibbs, J. T. (1992). Homicide and suicide in young black males: The Janus face of despair. In C. D. Llewelyn & R. J. Brown (Eds.), *The African-American male: A second emancipation* (pp. 15-26). New York: The National Urban League.

Gibbs, J. T., & Bankhead-Greene, T. (1996). *Joblessness and hopelessness: Black youth in south central Los Angeles.* Paper presented at the International Association of Social Workers Conference, Hong Kong, July 24-28, 1996.

Gibbs, J. T., & Fuery, D. (1994). Mental health and well-being of black women: Toward strategies of empowerment. *American Journal of Community Psychology, 22*(4), 559-582.

Gibbs, J. T., & Hines, A. M. (1989). Factors related to sex differences in suicidal behavior among black youth: Implications for intervention and research. *Journal of Adolescent Research, 4*(2), 152-172.

Gibbs, J., & Martin, W. (1964). *Status integration and suicide.* Eugene: University of Oregon Press.

Giddings, P. (1984). *When and where I enter: The impact of black women on race and sex in America.* New York: William Morrow.

Greene, B. (1994). African American women. In L. Comas-Diaz & B. Greene (Eds.), *Women of color: Integrating ethnic and gender identities in psychotherapy* (pp. 10-29). New York: Guilford Press.

Griffith, E. E., & Bell, C. C. (1989). Recent trends in suicide and homicide among blacks. *Journal of the American Medical Association, 262*, 2265-2269.

Heacock, D. R. (1990). Suicidal behavior in Black and Hispanic youth. *Psychiatric Annals, 20*(3), 134-142.

Heckler, M. (1985). *Report of the Secretary's Task Force on black and minority health.* Washington, DC: U.S. Department of Health and Human Services.

Hendin, H. (1969). Black suicide. *Archives of General Psychiatry, 21,* 407-422.
Hendin, H. (1978). Suicide: The psychosocial dimensions. *Suicide and Life-Threatening Behavior, 8*(2), 99-117.
Hickman, L. C. (1984). Descriptive differences between black and white suicide attempters. *Issues in Mental Health Nursing, 6,* 293-310.
Hill, R. (1972). *The strengths of Black families.* New York: Emerson Hall.
Howze, B. (1977). Suicide: Special reference to black women. *Journal of Non-White Concerns, 5,* 65-72.
Jackson, J. J. (1980). *Minorities and aging.* Belmont, CA: Wadsworth.
Kempton, T., & Forehand, R. L. (1992). Suicide attempts among juvenile delinquents: The contribution of mental health factors. *Behavior Research and Therapy, 30*(5), 537-541.
Kirk, A., & Zucker, R. (1979). Some sociopsychological factors in attempted suicide among urban Black males. *Suicide and Life-Threatening Behavior, 9,* 76-86.
Lester, D. (1990-91). Mortality from suicide and homicide for African-Americans in the U.S.A.: A regional analysis. *Omega: Journal of Death and Dying, 22*(3), 219-226.
Lester, D., & Anderson, D. (1992). Depression and suicidal ideation in African-American and Hispanic American high school students. *Psychological Reports, 71*(2), 618.
Lincoln, C. E. & Mamiya, L. (1990). *The Black church in the African American experience.* Durham, NC: Duke University Press.
Maris, R. W. (1995). Suicide prevention in adults (age 30-65). *Suicide and Life-Threatening Behavior, 25*(1), 171-179.
Martin, W. (1984). Religiosity and United States suicide rates, 1972-1978. *Journal of Clinical Psychology, 40,* 1166-1169.
Marzuk, P. M., Tardiff, K., Leon, A. C., Stajic, M., Morgan, E. B., & Mann, J. J. (1992). Prevalence of cocaine use among residents of New York City who committed suicide during a one-year period. *American Journal of Psychiatry, 149*(3), 371-375.
McAdoo, H. P. (Ed.) (1981). *Black families.* Beverly Hills, CA: Sage.
Meehan, P. J., Saltzman, L. E., & Sattin, R. W. (1991). Suicides among older United States residents: Epidemiologic characteristics and trends. *American Journal of Public Health, 81*(9), 1198-1200.
Minkler, M., & Roe, K. M. (1993). *Grandmothers as caregivers: Raising children of the crack cocaine epidemic.* Newbury Park, CA: Sage.
Molock, S. D., Kimbrough, R., Lacy, M. B., McClure, K. P., et al. (1994). Suicidal behavior among African-American college students: A preliminary study. *Journal of Black Psychology, 20*(2), 234-251.
Murphy, G. E., Wetzel, R. D., Robins, E., & McEvoy, L. (1992). Multiple risk factors predict suicide in alcoholism. *Archives of General Psychiatry, 49*(6), 459-463.
Myers, L. J. (1980). *Black women: Do they cope better?* Englewood Cliffs, NJ: Prentice Hall.
National Center for Health Statistics. (1994). *Vital Statistics of the United States, 1991*; vol. 2. Hyattsville, MD: Public Health Service.
Neigher, P. L., & Hopkins, R. W. (1988). Adolescent suicide: Character traits of high-risk teenagers. *Adolescence, 23,* 469-475.
Orfield, G. & Ashkinaze, C. (1991). *The closing door: Conservative policy and Black opportunity.* Chicago: University of Chicago Press.
Peck, D. L. (1983). "Official documentation" of the black suicide experience. *Omega: Journal of Death and Dying, 14,* 21-31.
Phillips, D. P., & Ruth, T. E. (1993). Adequacy of official suicide statistics for scientific research and public policy. *Suicide and Life-Threatening Behavior, 23*(4), 307-319.
Poussaint, A. (1977). Rising suicide rates among blacks. *Urban League Review, 3*(1), 22-30.
Proctor, C., & Groze, V. (1994). Risk factors for suicide among gay, lesbian and bi-sexual youths. *Social Work, 39*(5), 504-513.
Ramafedi, G., Farrow, J. A., & Deisher, R. W. (1991). Risk factors for attempted suicide in gay and bisexual youth. *Pediatrics, 87*(6), 869-875.
Rotheram-Borus, M. J. (1993). Suicidal behavior and risk factors among runaway youths. *American Journal of Psychiatry, 150*(1), 103-107.
Rotheram-Borus, M. J., Hunter, J., & Rosario, M. (1994). Suicidal behavior and gay-related stress among gay and bisexual male adolescents. *Journal of Adolescent Research, 9*(4), 498-508.
Rutledge, E. M. (1990). Suicide among black adolescents and young adults: A rising problem. In A. R. Stiffman & L. E. Davis (Eds.), *Ethnic issues in adolescent mental health* (pp. 339-351). Newbury Park, CA: Sage.
Seiden, R. (1982). Mellowing with age: Factors influencing the non-white suicide rate. *International Journal of Aging and Human Development, 13*(4), 265-284.
Shaffer, D., & Fisher, P. (1981). The epidemiology of suicide in children and young adolescents. *Journal of the American Academy of Child Psychiatry, 20,* 545-565.
Shaffer, D., Gould, M., & Hicks, R. C. (1994). Worsening suicide rate in black teenagers. *American Journal of Psychiatry, 151*(12), 1810-1812.
Stack, C. (1974). *All our kin: Strategies for survival in a black community.* New York: Harper and Row.
Summerville, M. B., Abbate, M. F., Siegel, A. M., Serravezza, J., et al. (1992). Psychopathology in urban female minority adolescents with suicide attempts. *Journal of the American Academy of Child and Adolescent Psychiatry, 31*(4), 663-668.
Summerville, M. B., Kaslow, N. J., Abbate, M. F., & Cronan, S. (1994). Psychopathology, family functioning, and cognitive style in urban adolescents with suicide attempts. *Journal of Abnormal Child Psychology, 22*(2), 221-235.
Swanson, W., & Breed, W. (1976). Black suicide in New Orleans. In E. S. Schneidman (Ed.), *Suicidology: Contemporary developments.* New York: Grune & Stratton.
Taylor, R. L. (Ed.), (1995). *African-American youth: Their social and economic status in the United States.* Westport, CT: Praeger.
Topol, P., & Resnikoff, M. (1982). Perceived peer and family relationships, hopelessness, and locus of

control as factors in adolescent suicide. *Suicide and Life-Threatening Behavior, 12,* 143-150.

Trautman, P. D., Rotherman-Borus, M. J., Dopkins, S., & Lewin, N. (1991). Psychiatric diagnoses in minority female adolescent suicide attempters. *Journal of the American Academy of Child and Adolescent Psychiatry, 30*(4), 617-622.

Vega, W. A., Gil, A., Warheit, G., Apospori, E., & Zimmerman, R. (1993). The relationship of drug use to suicide ideations and attempts among African-American, Hispanic and White non-Hispanic male adolescents. *Suicide and Life-Threatening Behavior, 23*(2), 110-119.

Walter, H. J., Vaughan, R. D., Armstrong, B., Krakoff, R. Y., et al. (1995). Sexual, assaultive, and suicidal behaviors among urban minority junior high school students. *Journal of the American Academy of Child and Adolescent Psychiatry, 34*(1), 78-80.

Warshauer, M., & Monk, M. (1978). Problems in suicide statistics for whites and blacks. *American Journal of Public Health, 68,* 383-388.

Wilson, M. (1981). Suicidal behavior: Toward an explanation of differences in female and male rates. *Suicide and Life-Threatening Behavior, 11,* 131-140.

Wilson, W. J. (1987). *The truly disadvantaged: The inner city, the underclass, and public policy.* Chicago: University of Chicago Press.

Wyche, K. F., & Rotheram-Borus, M. J. (1990). Suicide behavior among minority youth in the United States. In A. R. Stiffman & L. E. Davis (Eds.), *Ethnic issues in adolescent mental health* (pp. 323-338.) Newbury Park, CA: Sage.

9
Suicide in San Francisco, CA: A Comparison of Caucasian and Asian Groups, 1987–1994

Julia Shiang, EdD, PhD, Robert Blinn, PhD, Bruce Bongar, PhD, Boyd Stephens, MD, Donna Allison, PhD, and Alan Schatzberg, MD

Completed suicides in the city of San Francisco, California, were examined across all ages in the racial groups of Caucasians ($n = 798$) and Asians ($n = 124$) from 1987 to 1994. A comparison of Caucasians and Asians showed that there were differences between them in their rates across all age groups. The major findings are: (1) Caucasians predominately used gunshot to complete suicide whereas Asians predominately used hanging to complete suicide, (2) Asian women over the age of 85 have the highest rates across both groups and genders, (3) Asians, as compared to Caucasians, used fewer drugs and alcohol at time of death. Theoretical connections between differences in suicide and definition of the self, as influenced by culture, are discussed.

The empirical study of suicide is essential to determining effective prevention and treatment approaches for all groups in the United States. This paper focuses on the prevalence, method, gender, age group, and use of substances in suicide for two racial categories of people – Asians and Caucasians – in the city of San Francisco (S.F.), California, for a seven-year period (1987–1994).

The National Center for Health Statistics at the Centers for Disease Control and Prevention (Kachur, Potter, James, & Powell, 1995) reports different suicide rates across racial groups. Comparison across all male age groups showed that Native Americans have the highest rates, and then, in descending order, Whites, Blacks, and Asian/Pacific Islanders. In contrast, White females have the highest rates, followed by Native Americans, Asian/Pacific Islanders, and at the lowest rate, Blacks. Specific Asian data are also provided: the 1990 suicide rates reported for Asian males across all age groups indicate an overall rate of 8.8/100,000, with the highest rates at ages 15–24 (13.45/100,000), 75–84 (19.55/100,000), and 85+ (42.1/100,000). National rates for Asian females across all age groups indicate that they complete suicide at a rate of 3.4/100,000, with the highest rates at ages 55–64 (6.4/100,000), 75–84 (13.9/100,000), and 85+ (29.8/100,000). The predominant method used both among males and females was strangulation.

This study was designed to investigate completed suicides in the city of San Francisco with a particular focus on delineating the similarities and differences be-

Julia Shiang, EdD, PhD, is an Assistant Professor at Pacific Graduate School of Psychology and Lecturer at Stanford University School of Medicine. Robert Blinn, PhD, is at Blue Valley Mental Health Center. Bruce Bongar, PhD, is a Professor at Pacific Graduate School of Psychology and Consulting Professor at Stanford University School of Medicine. Boyd Stephens, MD, is Chief Medical Examiner; and Donna Allison, PhD, is Statistician and Data Analyst, at the Medical Examiner's Office, San Francisco. Alan Schatzberg, MD, is the Kenneth T. Norris, Jr., Professor and Chairman of the Department of Psychiatry and Behavioral Sciences at Stanford University School of Medicine. Please send all correspondence to the first author at PGSP, 935 East Meadow Dr., Palo Alto, CA 94303.

The authors would like to acknowledge the generous consultation of Dr. David Clark, Dr. Morton Silverman, Dr. Anita Greene, and Dr. Michelle Kalehzan. Data collection was completed with the help of Steven Barron, Loraine Van Tuyl, Toan Voung, and Jorge Wong. The study was funded, in part, by the American Suicide Foundation.

Suicide and Life-Threatening Behavior, Vol. 27(1), Spring 1997

tween Caucasian and Asian groups. The relatively high density of many racial groups in San Francisco provides us with a particularly suitable place to study suicide. According to the census data of 1990, the ratio of Asian to Caucasians is 1: 1.6 (210,876:337,118). The total population of the city is, of course, also made up of other ethnic groups–African Americans, Hispanics, Native Americans, and others.

Findings from the study would help inform the development of treatment programs. For example, if the patterns of completing suicide in the two groups are more or less similar, then the findings would provide further evidence to support a common conceptualization of suicide risk. Presently available prevention and intervention programs that are based on Western-based models of mental health could thus be imported into immigrant Asian communities with support for their expected effectiveness. If significant differences between the groups emerge, then the theory of difference between the independence and interdependence definition of self might be supported and, furthermore, concerns about the successful applicability of aspects of Western-based models of care with Asians in the United States would be raised; new models of intervention would be required.

In this paper we address the following three questions.

1. Do Caucasians and Asians show similar rates across age group? Is there a difference between the groups in the geriatric population?
2. Are there other differences (in age, method, use of substances, etc.) between the groups?
3. Are there specific recommendations that can be made for intervention programs in San Francisco and other urban settings?

PRIOR STUDIES

Few studies have examined completed suicides among Chinese Americans, a subgroup of Asians, whose heritage was based in China (presently the People's Republic of China), Hong Kong, Taiwan, and other Asian countries. Borne (1973) focused on Chinese Americans in the period 1952–1968 in San Francisco and found that the rate for completed suicides over all age groups was 27.9/100,000. This was comparable to the general population rate of 27.5/100,000 for the city of S.F. at that time. However, the rates of suicide among Chinese Americans, age 55 and older, was dramatically higher at 50+/100,000 than the average for the population of the entire city. Rates for Asian females rose from ages 65–74 (35.1/100,000) to ages 75+ (43.3/100,000). Rates for Asian men were generally higher, with the highest rate in the 65–74 age group (63/100,000). This study suggests that the two racial groups (Caucasians and Asians) are not very different except in the age group above 50 years.

In another study, Yu, Chang, Liu, and Fernandez (1986) studied national data for youth (ages 15–24) among Chinese Americans. They found that in 1970, the national age-adjusted rate for Chinese Americans in the 15- to 24-year-old age group was 2.98/100,000. By 1980, the rate had more than doubled (6.39/100,000). This suggests that this particular population is at risk.

These data suggest that varying cultural practices and behaviors may have an impact on suicidal behavior, particularly for the geriatric population. Past research in the areas of anthropology (Geertz, 1983), cross-cultural studies (Bond, 1986), psychiatric anthropology (Kleinman, 1988), and ethnic minority studies (Padilla, Wagatsuma, & Lindholm, 1985; Sue & Zane, 1994) as well as recent research in the area of cultural psychology (Markus & Kitayama, 1994; Shweder, 1991) suggest that cultural practices are much more important than previously thought in determining day-to-day behaviors, including the patterns that a person chooses to complete suicide.

Recent work in the area of cultural psychology examines the multiple and systematic ways in which cultural beliefs, values, and the resultant differences in the construal of the self in the world create and maintain specific psychological processes (Markus & Kitayama, 1994). Beliefs concerning death, its meanings, and attributions made in the act of suicide, are thus formed, to a large degree, by cultural practices. One of the ways in which Western and Asian cultures have been contrasted is through research that focuses on the definition of the self. Research findings indicate that Western cultures are largely based on belief systems that foster independence; the enhancement of the self is of primary importance. In contrast, Asian cultures emphasize interdependence or interconnectedness, and the self is therefore viewed as being a part of a group; the needs of the individual are not regarded as being as important as the needs of the group, especially in a public setting. Asian cultural groups are conceptualized as having a "core psychological tendency" (Markus & Kitayama, 1994, p. 106) that is focused on relationships or interconnectedness. Good feelings about the self may derive

> from realizing the approach to selfhood required by . . . interdependent cultures. Indeed, good feelings may be a function of good social relationships (i.e., fitting-in, belonging, maintaining harmony in one's relationships, occupying one's proper place, engaging in appropriate action) while at the same time regulating one's inner personal thoughts and feelings so as to ensure interdependence. (Markus & Kitayama, 1994, p. 106)

The ramification of this difference is that death in Western cultures would be largely thought of as a independent act whereas suicide in Asian cultures would be an act thought of in the context of relationships. Support for this view comes from the differences in the typical response to a suicide in these cultures. In Western cultures, the question asked is: "Why? Why did this happen." The perspective is that the individual has made a "choice" to commit suicide. In Asian culture the question often asked after a suicide is: "Who caused this death? Who drove this person to suicide?"

METHOD

Study Population

Data for 922 cases were collected from July 1, 1987 to June 30, 1994. The total number of Caucasians who completed suicide during this time period was 798; the total number of Asians was 124 (see Table 1 for sample characteristics).

The data were obtained in cooperation with the Medical Examiner's office of San Francisco County, who routinely documents the completed suicides in the city of San Francisco. Official records include information on age, gender, race, and method of suicide. Postmortem tissue specimens obtained at time of death were tested for the presence or absence of alcohol, and the office has the capability to test for over 100 prescription medications, illicit drugs, over-the-counter medications, poisons, and other substances in the bloodstream at time of death.

Variable Definitions

Variables that were to be of interest were: age, gender, method, and use of substances at time of death. These were extracted from the information provided by the Medical Examiner's Office. The decisions of the office related to these variables were used as documented.

The racial designations of the individuals used in this study were accepted as designated by the Medical Examiner's

TABLE 1
Characteristics of the Sample

	Caucasians	Asians
Sample size (*n*)	798	124
Age range (years)	13–95	17–96
Mean age	48	53
Female (*n*)	183	45
Males (*n*)	615	77

Office in San Francisco. Possible designations of race were: Unknown, White, Black, Hispanic, Oriental, and Asian (with the possibility of 7 separate ethnic designations, including Pacific Islander). When information from the deceased's family or friends was not available, the personnel from the Medical Examiner's Office made the racial designation. Identification was made by reference to either surname or facial features. We acknowledge that there are inherent problems with the use of surname because of marriage, adoption of names, etc. With regard to facial recognition, our understanding is that this office has, in comparison to most offices around the country, had a greater than average share in identifying Asians due to the fact that the population of Asians in San Francisco is relatively large.

For example, the statistics provided by the National Center for Injury Prevention and Control (Kachur, et al., 1995), to their credit, clearly state that racial categories are not consistently recorded on death certificate information from which they gather information. Their solution in reporting information on race is to employ the following classifications: White, Non-Hispanic, Black, Native American, Hispanic, Asian/Pacific Islander, and "other." In general, the category of "other" has been made up of a composite of many races that excludes Whites and Blacks but includes many diverse cultures and ethnic groups such as Asians, Hispanics, Native Americans, and so on. The categorization of people into one large racial group may actually reflect many diverse ethnic groups; for example, Caucasians are made up of diverse and varied groups from the Irish to the Italian. Asians, as a race, include people whose heritage is based in such diverse geographic locations such as China, Thailand, Vietnam, India, Taiwan, etc. Within each geographic location there are many ethnic groups who share beliefs and practices with other Asians, and yet recognizably distinctly different cultural beliefs and practices exist in each as well. For example, culture-bound syndromes such as *koro* of Malaysian origin or *shen-k'uei* of Taiwan exist only in certain communities. We acknowledge that these racial designations are less than perfect. The larger issue of designation of race is a difficult and thorny one; it is an issue currently being debated in the fields that study culture and race (Yee, Fairchild, Weizmann, & Wyatt, 1993). A more thorough discussion is not possible here. Although these difficulties present a limitation to the findings of the study, we believe that clarification of decision making is the best approach for the eventual determination of a uniform standard for using racial designations as a variable for scientific study.

For the purposes of this study, we relabeled the designations as follows: (1) the Oriental, Asian, and Pacific Islander categories were collapsed and designated as "Asian." (2) Designations of the category of Whites were uniformly relabeled as "Caucasians." In discussion with colleagues, we decided to parallel the information available through the label; the term "Caucasian" signifies a Euro-American heritage.

Rates and Statistical Analyses

Age-adjusted suicide rates per 100,000 were calculated using the same age groupings as employed by the Centers for Disease Control and Prevention. Data on completed suicides were available for the complete years of 1988 through 1993. Population figures for racial groups in San Francisco were obtained from the 1990 Census of Population for California (U.S. Department of Commerce, Bureau of the Census, 1992). Rates were calculated by determining a yearly average number of deaths based on the incidence of suicide found in San Francisco. The incidence per 100,000 for San Francisco was determined with the age-specific population figures of San Francisco for 1990.

Frequencies for each variable were tabulated and subjected to appropriate statistical analyses. Chi-square analyses were used to determine levels of significance.

RESULTS

The major findings are summarized as follows:

1. Caucasian females are at greatest risk in the middle age range (45–54) whereas Asian females are at greatest risk in the old old age range (85+).
2. Caucasian males are at greatest risk in the old old age range (85+) whereas Asian males are at greater risk somewhat earlier (75–84), and this increased risk continues into old-old age.
3. The ratio of female to male suicides among Caucasians is 1:3, whereas the ratio for Asians is closer to 1:2.
4. Caucasians generally use gunshot whereas Asians generally use hanging to complete suicide.
5. Caucasians generally use alcohol and abusive drugs at time of death whereas Asians generally use drugs at time of death.
6. Asians show significantly lower psychotropic drug use at time of death than do Caucasians.

Suicide Rates Among Caucasians and Asians, 1988–1993

The calculated rates of suicide per 100,000 population for the San Francisco sample, adjusted for age-specific population figures, showed that Caucasians have consistently higher rates than Asians across all age groups (see Fig. 1).

Suicide Rates and Gender Differences

Caucasian and Asian female rates for the total sample were, respectively, 19.49/100,000 and 14.45/100,000 (see Fig. 2). The higher rates for Caucasians as compared to Asians held across all age groups with the exception of age 85+, where Asian females exceeded Caucasian females at a ratio of 2.7 to 1. Caucasian female peak at age 45–54 (30/100,000), then dip downward but rise slightly at age 85+ (27/100,000). Asians had an overall lower rate except in old age, where they exhibited a sharp spike in their rate in the 85+ age group (67/100,000).

A comparison of males, on the other hand, showed that Caucasian males have an overall rate of 68.25/100,000 whereas the Asian males have an overall rate of 18.45/100,000. A comparison across age groups (see Fig. 3) showed that the pattern of completed suicides for Caucasian males peaked in the 45–54 age group (70/100,000), and then again in the 75–84 and 85+ age groups (83/100,000 and 123/100,000, respectively). For Asian males the rate was lower across all ages, except in the 75–84 age group (50/100,000).

Figures 4 and 5 presents the ratios of females to males for both groups. Caucasian females to males showed a 1:3 ratio in completed suicides across all age groups. This was not so for the Asian sample. In the middle age groups, the ratio of completed suicides for females to males was 1:2; at age 65–74 it was almost 1:1; then at ages 75–84, was 1:3; but then surprisingly, at age 85+, the Asian female-to-male ratio was again 1:2. In other words, 2 females over the age of 85 completed suicide for every Asian male of the same age.

Statistical Comparisons Across Racial Groups

Significant differences were also found between Caucasians and Asians for type of method used to complete suicide ($\chi^2 = 13.04$, $df = 4$, $p = .011$), the presence or absence of ETOH ($\chi^2 = 7.82$, $df = 1$, $p = .005$) at time of death, intoxication at time of death ($\chi^2 = 17.46$, $df = 1$, $p = .000$), and the use of drugs ($\chi^2 = 8.86$, $df = 1$, $p = .002$) at time of death (Table 2). We examine these findings in more depth below.

Method and Age Group. Significant differences were found in the method ($\chi^2 = 13.04$, $df = 4$, $p = .011$) used by Caucasians and Asians across all age groups to

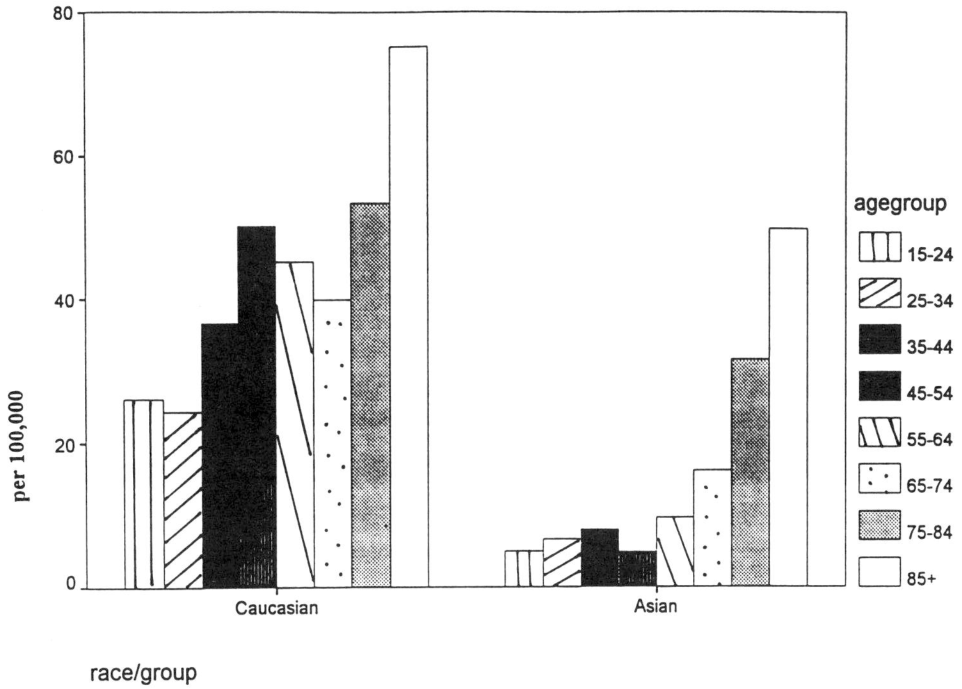

Figure 1. Age-specific suicide rates in San Francisco, CA, 1986–1993. $N = 922$, Caucasian and Asian.

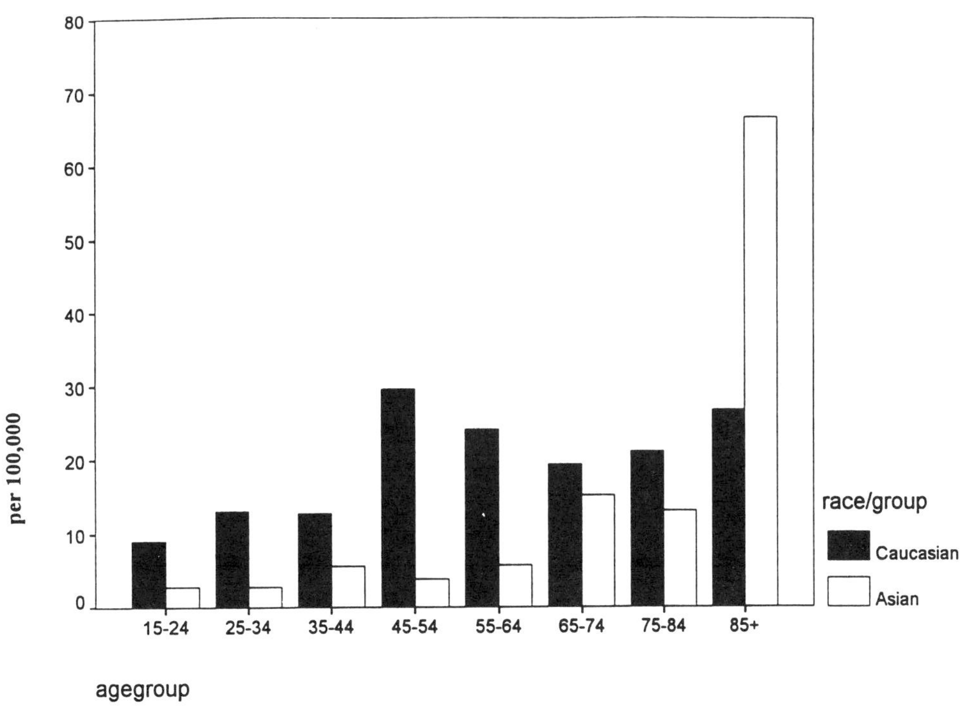

Figure 2. Age-specific suicide rates for females. Caucasian ($n = 183$) and Asian ($n = 45$).

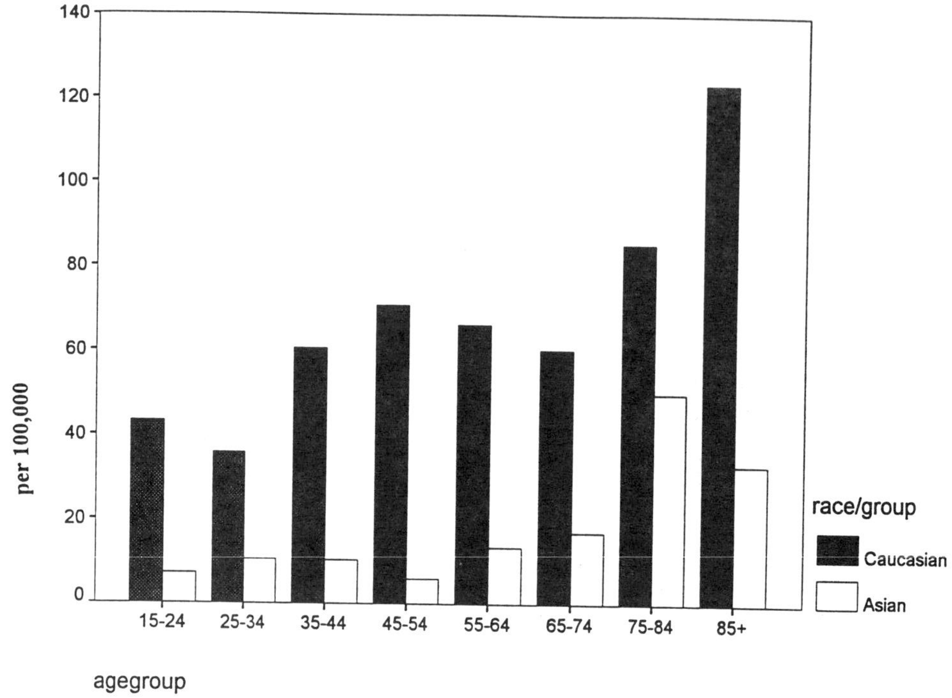

Figure 3. Age-specific suicide rates for males. Caucasian (n = 615) and Asian (n = 77).

complete suicide among the methods of gunshot, hanging, jumping, overdose, and other (includes asphyxia, stabbing, cutting, CO poisoning, drowning, ingestion, burns, and a combination of methods). Caucasians predominately used gunshot whereas the Asians predominately used hanging when they are compared across age groups. Figure 6 presents the percentage of completed suicides by category of method and race.

Use of Alcohol and Intoxication at Time of Death. A comparison of use of alcohol among Caucasians and Asians shows significant differences in the use of alcohol at time of death ($\chi^2 = 7.82$, $df = 1$, $p = .005$). Thirty-one percent of all Caucasians used alcohol at time of death whereas only 8% of all Asians used alcohol at time of death. To set an intoxication level, we used the standard criteria used by California police (>0.08% blood alcohol level). With this criterion significant differences were found across the racial designations ($\chi^2 = 17.46$, $df = 1$, $p = .000$); 22.5% of Caucasians were found to be intoxicated at death whereas 6% of Asians were found to be intoxicated.

DISCUSSION

The present study expands the information now available on completed suicide in an urban context where the proportion of Caucasian and Asian population allows for a reasonable comparison. We have shown that striking differences exist between Caucasians and Asians in their patterns of suicide across the basic variables of age group, method, and use of substances at time of death.

How do we understand the differences between Caucasian and Asian patterns of completing suicide? Differences in life patterns, life expectations, and access to means of completing suicide would all provide further understanding of these patterns. Unfortunately, the data available to

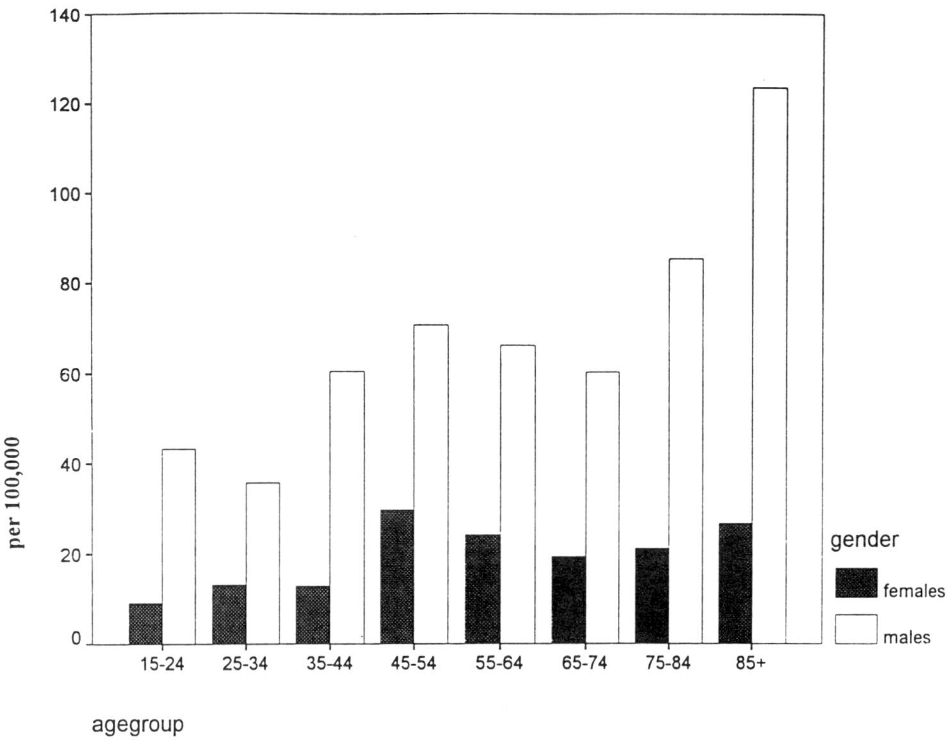

Figure 4. Age-specific suicide rates for Caucasians, by gender (n = 798).

us did not allow for these types of comparisons.

The question of whether cultural practices and differences in the construal of the self help us to understand these differences can be considered, albeit indirectly. There are some compelling similarities between the general patterns of suicide as practiced in Asia and the patterns of suicide among Asians in San Francisco. We are interested in considering whether these patterns of suicide suggest a self-construal that is more interconnected than independent.

There are two specific Asian cultural practices that help provide an understanding of the suicide pattern for Asians in San Francisco. First, in Asia, the elderly are revered; old age is explicitly a time when adult children provide care for elderly in return for the care they received as children. In the United States the predominate ethos is that the elderly should not be a burden to their adult children; they should maintain independence as long as possible. Over the past decade many elderly Asian parents have emigrated to the United States to live with their now-adult children expecting to receive care from their adult children. But as their children adopt "American ways," they often choose not to care for their elderly in the ways that would be expected by traditional Asian norms. Elderly are left without the support systems and resources they believe is their "right." The reality for the elderly parents is that they don't see their children very often; their expectations of being revered, much less taken care of, are not actualized. Furthermore their views of themselves as "good parents" who raised filial children are now shattered and they feel shamed (Shiang, 1986). This would be especially true for elderly women, now widowed, who determine their own self-worth in terms of harmonious relationships with adult children, compared to men, who derive self-

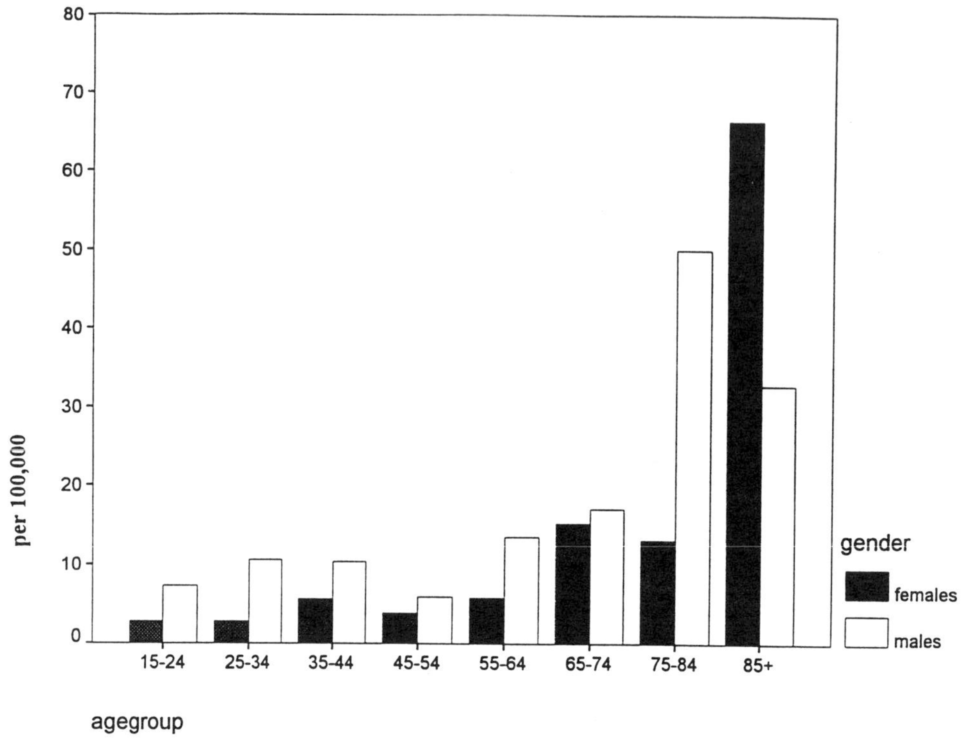

Figure 5. Age-specific suicide rates for Asians, by gender (n = 124).

worth from instrumental achievements—elderly women have few options when their own children ignore them. The high level of discrepancy between expectations and actual practices puts the elderly at greater risk for suicide. It may be for these reasons that Asian elderly are at higher risk of suicide.

The choice of method can also be understood in terms of cultural construals of self as interconnected. It is clear that hanging is still the preferred method used in choosing to die for most Asians. Why would Asians choose hanging as the predominant method for completing suicide?

Some information related to Chinese beliefs and behaviors concerning suicide may be useful, as the Chinese make up the largest proportion of all Asians in San Francisco. We would, however, fully expect that a person from another Asian culture (e.g., Thailand, Malaysia, Japan) to attribute different specific meanings to the act of suicide even though their self-construal may be based on more or less the same motivation of interconnectedness.

In traditional China respect was given

TABLE 2
Comparison of Asian and Caucasian Groups Across Variables

	Suicide (n)	Chi-square	df	p value
Method × Race	891	13.04	4	.0110
Alcohol present × Race	921	7.82	1	.0050
Intoxication × Race	912	17.46	1	.0000
Drugs used × Race	870	8.86	1	.0020

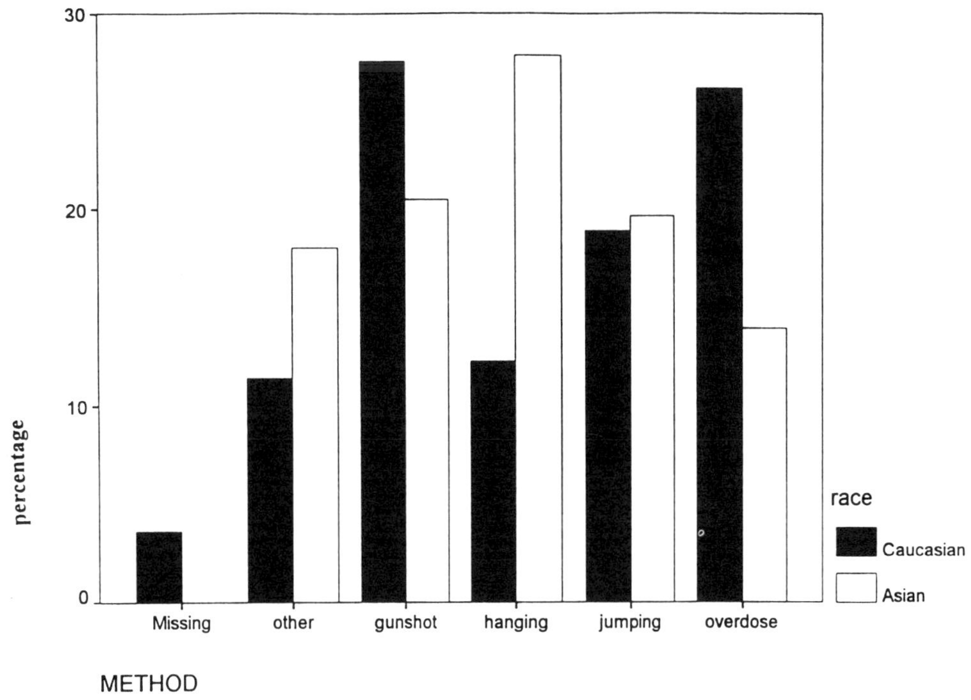

Figure 6. Percentages of completed suicides, method by race. $N = 891$, chi-square = 13.04, $df = 4$, $p = .011$.

for those who committed suicide out of loyalty to a person or the state (Hsieh & Spence, 1980). Asian society sees the act of suicide as an interpersonal act. Suicide takes place in a context–defined by both the individual and the group. In terms of societal needs, the assignment of an interpersonal motivation for causing the act allows the group to move the emphasis away from concerns about personal misery. The individual person and his or her motivations are secondary to the overall needs of the group to maintain smooth interpersonal relations. At the same time, in traditional views, the act of suicide was seen as purposeful and its intention could also be to send a message to those left behind. The person who "caused" the suicide could then be admonished for his or her shameful conduct so that the community could teach the person a moral lesson. Suicide could also act as a vehicle for revenge; the belief is that the restless spirit of the deceased would return to haunt the living. Farberow (1975) was one of the first researchers who examined the influence of Confucianism, Buddhism, and Taoism on suicide; with these belief systems the meaning of suicide is less individualistic than it is familial.

These belief systems are expressed in behavioral patterns as well; the Chinese predominantly used hanging as a method of suicide in traditional China. Bourne (1973) stated that in traditional China,

> the ghosts of those who die by hanging return[ed] to torment the living in a particularly persistent and vicious manner. Committing suicide by hanging . . . carried the implication of great anger and resentment by the victim towards those in his or her own immediate environment. For the subjugated women in traditional Chinese society who could not express their anger openly, dying by hanging was a means of achieving final and lasting vengeance. While this method is probably rarely, if ever considered consciously by the victims, it has perhaps established a cultural precedence for selecting hanging as a method for suicide which is unknowingly passed on from one generation to the another. (pp. 747–748)

The predominant use of hanging in this sample may be seen as an interpersonal act. The use of hanging, with its specific cultural interpretations, emphasizes belonging and community. This suggests that this cultural belief system still endures and has been resistant to change even in the face of living in a new culture.

LIMITATIONS OF THE STUDY

There are a number of methodological concerns that influence any study conducted with data based on death certificates or medical examiner's reports. Methodological concerns include inaccuracies in reporting the incidence of suicide as well as the underreporting of the population in the census. These would influence the calculation of the rate of suicide. Concerns about recordkeeping and obtaining accurate demographic information from the people who were present at the site of death are considerations that would apply to any data set. Local events like the 1989 San Francisco earthquake and the resulting shutdown of the main highway artery that leads to Chinatown's business district would also have had an impact on the economic health of the community but are difficult to tie directly to incidence of suicide based on the data available to us.

Second, we are unable to consider the impact of the environment and cohort effects of the sample. San Francisco shares with many other settings the same set of advantages and disadvantages of urban living. The advantage to this study of the large numbers of races available for comparison living in the city also serves to contribute to the numerous lifestyles and cultural practices that are unique to San Francisco. The city is also well known for its relatively large gay community. The findings related to method may also be due to cohort effects; for example, Caucasians ages 55–64 used gunshot less than other ages. This group were in their 20s at the time of the Vietnam war; the impact of surviving a war might influence their attitudes toward using guns. Asians in the 45-year-old age group also showed a lower rate; they were born at the time of the Communist Revolution in Mainland China and their families experienced a great deal of upheaval and chaos. These historical events can influence one's attitude about the meaning of life and the method used to end one's life. Information related to the effects of these factors was not available to us in this study but should be considered for possible contributions to cohort effects.

Information was not available on the subjects' access to lethal means of ending one's life (guns) or on the accessibility of substances. However, it is commonly understood that firearms are readily available in the United States; whether they are more available to people living in San Francisco is difficult to determine. There are, of course, two bridges, the Golden Gate Bridge and the Bay Bridge, which cumulatively have been the site of over 100 suicides in the course of their histories. Jumping (from buildings, from bridges, etc.) was the fourth highest method used (20% for each group) for completing suicide in this sample; in the national data jumping is grouped with "other methods" and accounts for only 6% of the total.

TREATMENT RECOMMENDATIONS

We suggest that physicians, usually the first and only contact with health professionals, who are treating elderly Asians pay greater attention to the possibility of suicide, especially among elderly Asian women. The stereotype of the frail, small, quiet, and passive elderly Asian woman is belied in the finding that they exhibit some of the highest rates of completed suicide.

Second, treatment programs for mental health with Caucasians must focus on both alcohol and drug use patterns whereas Asians should focus more on the use of drugs. Caucasians were also found to be intoxicated (>0.08% blood level) four times more often than Asians; Asians were using drugs 22% of the time at the time of their deaths.

We suggest than an understanding of culturally based practices are essential to understanding specific suicide patterns and the factors involved in increased risk of specific age groups. The programs that are presently based on Western models of mental health may not be effective for the prevention and reduction of suicide risk for Asians. To be effective, the cultural practices that endure in the face of migration must be considered an essential part of developing treatment programs.

REFERENCES

Bond, M. H. (Ed.). (1986). *The psychology of the Chinese people.* New York: Oxford University Press.

Bourne, P. G. (1973). Suicide among Chinese in San Francisco. *American Journal of Public Health, 8*(63), 744-750.

U.S. Department of Commerce, Bureau of the Census. (1995). Census of Population for California, 1990. Washington, DC: U.S. Government Printing Office.

Farberow, N. L. (1975). *Suicide in different cultures.* Baltimore: University Park Press.

Geertz, C. (1973). *The interpretation of cultures.* New York: Basic Books.

Geertz, C. (1983). *Local knowledge: Further essays in interpretative anthropology.* New York: Basic Books.

Hsieh, A. C. K., & Spence, J. (1980). Suicide and the family in pre-modern Chinese society. In A. Kleinman & T. Y. Lin (Eds.), *Normal and abnormal behavior in Chinese society.* The Netherlands: D. Reidel.

Kachur, S. P., Potter, L. B., James, S. B., & Powell, K. E. (1995). *Suicide in the United States, 1980–1992: Violence surveillance summary series, 1.* Atlanta, GA: Centers for Disease Control and Prevention, National Center for Injury Prevention and Control.

Kleinman, A. (1988). *The illness narratives: Suffering, healing, and the human condition.* New York: Basic Books.

Markus, H., & Kitayama, S. (1994). The cultural construction of self and emotion: Implications for social behavior. In S. Kitayama & H. Markus (Eds.), *Emotion and culture: Empirical studies of mutual influence* (pp. 89-130). Washington, DC: American Psychological Association.

Padilla, A., Wagatsuma, Y., & Lindholm, K. (1985). Acculturation and personality as predictors of stress in Japanese and Japanese-Americans. *Journal of Social Psychology, 125,* 295-305.

Shiang, J. (1986). "Heart" and self in old age: A Chinese model. In M. White & S. Pollack (Eds.), *The cultural transition: Human experience and social transformation in the Third World and Japan* (pp. 211-239). Boston: Routledge & Kegan Paul.

Shweder, R. A. (1991). *Thinking through cultures: Expeditions in cultural psychology.* Cambridge, MA: Harvard University Press.

Shweder, R. A., & LeVine, R. A. (Eds.). (1984). *Culture theory: Essays on mind, self, and emotion.* New York: Cambridge University Press.

Sue, S., & Zane, N. (1994). Research in psychotherapy with culturally diverse populations. In A. E. Bergin & S. L. Garfield (Eds.), *Handbook of psychotherapy and behavior change* (pp. 664-700). New York: Wiley.

U.S. Department of Commerce (1992). Economics and Statistics Administration. Bureau of the Census, 1990, CP-1-6.

Yee, A., Fairchild, H. H., Weizmann, F., & Wyatt, G. E. (1993). Addressing psychology problems with race. *American Psychologist, 48,* 1132-1140.

Yu, E., Chang, C., Liu, W., & Fernandez, M. (1986). *Suicide among Asian-American youth.* Report of the Secretary's Task Force on Youth Suicide. Washington, DC: U.S. Government Printing Office.

10
Suicidality Among Acculturating Mexican Americans: Current Knowledge and Directions for Research

Joseph D. Hovey and Cheryl A. King

Despite the dramatic increase in Mexican-American immigration over the past two decades, the acculturative experience and its relationship to suicide risk have received little attention within the field of suicidology. This paper summarizes findings from community-based studies that have explored suicide and risk factors among immigrant and Mexican-American groups, and suggests directions for future research. Most of these studies have been epidemiologic, and relatively few have addressed risk and protective factors within well-defined acculturating groups. Further study of the full continuum of suicidal thoughts and behaviors that examines precise cultural risk factors, and uses methodologies that combine quantitative and qualitative data, may improve our understanding of suicide risk among acculturating Mexican Americans.

> I don't know how my future will be because sometimes I feel as if the world was standing on its head and as if day to day I become sick and my head hurts. Rejection from those I love hurts. I feel as if I don't matter. I think my future will worsen, each day a bit more. . . . I don't know if it will be better. I don't know and I am not interested in knowing. Life for me is not worth anything now, nor will it ever. . . . (17-year-old male immigrant of Mexican descent) (Hovey & King, 1996, p. 1189)

The thought that suicide may stem from the lack of meaningful social interactions and close relationships within the community dates back to Durkheim (1897/1951). According to Durkheimian thought, "anomie" sets in and individuals are at a higher risk for suicide when the accustomed relationship between the individual and his or her society is shattered. This may occur when an individual migrates to a new country. In the new country an individual may feel pulled between the values of his or her ethnic group and that of the mainstream society. Caught in this state, certain individuals may experience heightened levels of psychological distress. This suggests that—during the acculturative process—immigrants may be at an increased risk for suicidal ideation and behavior.

Acculturative stress is a term currently used (e.g., Berry & Kim, 1988; Padilla, Cervantes, Maldonado, & Garcia, 1988; Williams & Berry, 1991) to describe the stress that directly results from, and has its source in the acculturative process. According to Williams and Berry (1991), acculturative stress may result in a particular set of emotions and behaviors including depression and anxiety, feelings of marginality and alienation, heightened psychosomatic symptoms, and identity confusion.

MODEL OF ACCULTURATIVE STRESS

Berry and Kim (1988) and Williams and Berry (1991) present a conceptual framework for studying the acculturative process and its relationship to mental health.

Joseph D. Hovey is with the Department of Psychology, University of Michigan. Cheryl A. King is with the Department of Psychiatry and Psychology, University of Michigan. Address correspondence concerning this article to Joseph D. Hovey, Department of Psychology, University of Michigan, 525 E. University, Ann Arbor, MI 48109-1109. E-mail: joehovey@umich.edu

Suicide and Life-Threatening Behavior, Vol. 27(1), Spring 1997

Their model identifies the cultural and psychological variables that may govern the relationship between acculturation and mental health. These include social support found within the new community; immediate and extended family support networks; socioeconomic status (SES), including work-status changes and specific characteristics of SES such as education and employment; premigration variables such as adaptive functioning (self-esteem, coping ability, psychiatric status), knowledge of the new language and culture, and motives for the move (voluntary versus involuntary); cognitive attributes such as attitudes toward acculturation (positive or negative) and expectations toward the future; and the nature of the larger society – that is, the degree of tolerance for, and acceptance of cultural diversity (multicultural versus assimilationist) within the mainstream society.

These variables may serve as "buffers" in the reduction of acculturative stress. Acculturating individuals with relatively high levels of family and social support may, for example, experience less acculturative stress than individuals without the same support. It is important to note that there is great variation in the amount of acculturative stress experienced by acculturating individuals. As Williams and Berry (1991, p. 634) state, the acculturative experience may eventually "enhance one's life chances and mental health or virtually destroy one's ability to carry on." One's acculturative outcome depends on the individual and group factors that moderate the acculturative process.

As shown in Figure 1, we have extended Williams and Berry's (1991) acculturative stress model to include possible *consequences* of heightened levels of acculturative stress. More specifically, we have suggested (Hovey & King, 1996) that the acculturative experience leads to varying levels of acculturative stress, and that elevated levels of acculturative stress may result in significant levels of depressive symptoms and suicidal ideation. Figure 1 illustrates this connection and lists the factors that possibly moderate levels of acculturative stress, depression, and suicidal ideation. The broken arrows represent influences that are probabilistic rather than deterministic.

SUICIDALITY WITHIN IMMIGRANT POPULATIONS

Scant attention has been given to the study of suicidality within immigrant populations. Moreover, those studies that do involve immigrant populations (e.g., Boor, 1981; Lester, 1989; Stack, 1981a, 1981b; Trovato, 1986a, 1986b) have usually focused on immigrants in a general sense, not on immigrants of specific ethnic groups, and have focused on completed suicide rate as the variable of study, rather than the continuum of suicidal thoughts and behaviors.

As an example of such a study, Trovato (1986a) examined suicide mortality within a data set consisting of several ethnic–immigrant groups in Canada (English–Welsh, American Scottish, Irish, German, Italian, Portuguese, other foreign born). He evaluated three dimensions of immigration–ethnicity: the assimilation thesis, which supposes that the greater the degree of social assimilation among immigrant–ethnic groups, the greater the suicide rate; the ethnic community integration explanation, which predicts that immigrant–ethnic groups with strong levels of community cohesiveness reveal reduced suicide rates; and the socioeconomic hypothesis, which states that immigrant–ethnic groups with greater socioeconomic levels reveal lower suicide rates. Analyzing the immigrant–ethnic groups together as a whole, Trovato conducted a factor analysis on aggregated social demographic characteristics and a consequent multiple regression analysis (on the factors corresponding to the three dimensions of immigration–ethnicity). He found some support for the assimilation and ethnic community integration hypotheses.

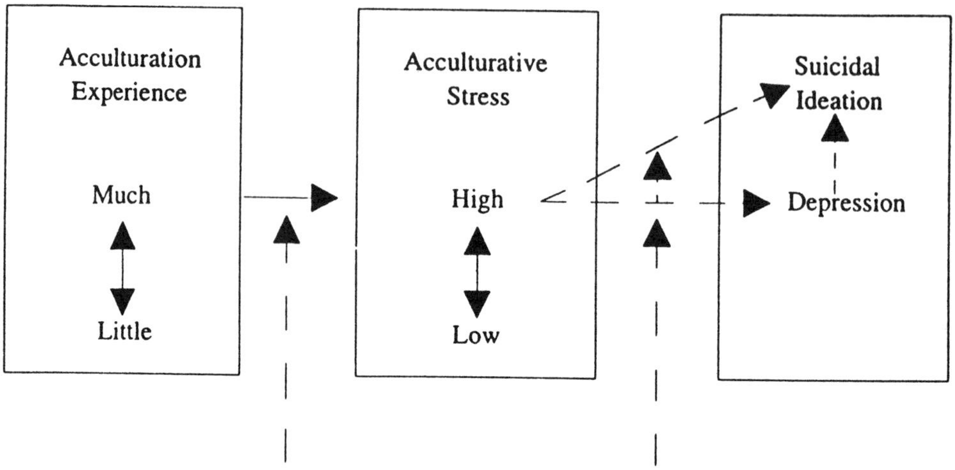

Variables Moderating The Relationships Between Acculturation, Acculturative Stress, Depression, And Suicidal Ideation

Family Cohesiveness: Family intactness and family functioning

Social Support: Access to social network and perceived effectiveness of support

Socioeconomic Status: Includes work-status changes

Premigration Adaptive Functioning: Includes self-esteem; coping ability; psychiatric status

Prior Knowledge of the New Language and Culture

Motives for the Move: Voluntary versus involuntary; internal versus external

Cognitive Variables: Attitudes toward acculturation; expectancies toward future; plans

Age at Immigration: Less stressful adaptation is expected with movement prior to age 12

Generation in New Community: Less stress expected with later generations

Degree of Cultural Pluralism within New Community: Multicultural ideology within community; acceptance of the specific culture within community

Figure 1. Model of acculturative stress, depression, and suicidal ideation.

SUICIDALITY AMONG MEXICAN AMERICANS

When looking at suicidality within the more specific immigrant–ethnic population of Mexican Americans, we again find little research. There are only a handful of studies exploring suicidality within the Mexican-American population. Most of these studies concentrate on adults. As examples, in a pair of community-based studies, Sorenson and Golding (1988a, 1988b) examined lifetime rates of suicidal ideation and suicide attempts among Latinos and non-Latino Whites. In the first study (Sorenson & Golding, 1988a), Mexican Americans born in Mexico revealed significantly lower age- and gender-adjusted lifetime rates of suicidal ideation (4.5%) than Mexican Americans born in the United States (13.0%), who revealed significantly lower rates than non-Latino Whites born in the United States (19.2%). Adjusted rates of suicide attempt were lowest among Mexican Americans born in Mexico (1.6%) and higher among both Mexican Americans (4.8%) and non-Latino Whites (4.4%) born in the United States. In the second study (Sorenson & Golding, 1988b), fewer Latinos (of which 87% were Mexican American) reported suicidal ideation (8.8% vs. 18.9%) and suicide attempts (3.2% vs. 5.1%) than non-Latino Whites.

Concerning suicide mortality, Smith, Mercy, and Warren (1985) compared suicide rates among Anglos and Latinos (of which 86% were Mexican American) in five southwestern states and found that, for all ages, the suicide rate for Latinos (9.0) in the area was less than that for Anglos (19.2). This discrepancy between groups, however, was less for adolescents (ages 15–19), as the suicide rate for Latino adolescents was 9.0 compared to 11.9 for Anglo adolescents. Suicides, moreover, occurred at a younger age for Latinos (32.9% under age 25) than for Anglos (17.3% under age 25). Anatore and Loya (1973), Hatcher and Hatcher (1975), and Hoppe and Martin (1986) also found that suicide rates for Mexican Americans declined with age. This pattern contrasts to the pattern typically found among both Anglos and individuals in Mexico, and thus suggests that suicide among Mexican Americans is more of a youthful phenomena.

As alluded to, very few studies (Hovey & King, 1996; Loya, 1976; Swanson, Linskey, Quintero-Salinas, Pumariega, & Holzer, 1992) have investigated suicidality among Mexican-American adolescents. Swanson et al. (1992) explored suicidal ideation, depressive symptoms, and drug use in a sample of Mexican and Mexican-American adolescents (ages 11–19) attending school in six border cities in Texas and neighboring Mexico. In comparison to the Mexican adolescents, the Mexican-American adolescents reported higher rates of current suicidal ideation (23.4 vs. 11.6%), depressive symptoms (48.1% vs. 39.4% scored above 16 on the Center for Epidemiologic Studies Depression Scale, which constitutes the scale's cutoff for determining caseness), and illicit drug use (21% vs. 5%). To explore the relationship between variables, the authors utilized logistic regression analyses and found a strong linkage between depressive symptoms, drug use, and suicidal ideation within adolescents of both countries.

Hovey and King (1996) explored the relationship between acculturative stress, depressive symptoms, and suicidal ideation in a sample of immigrant and second generation Latino-American (87% Mexican–American) adolescents. One fourth of the adolescents reported critical levels of depression and suicidal ideation, which were correlated positively with acculturative stress ($p < .01$ and $p < .001$, respectively). The authors used multiple regression analyses to explore the best predictors of elevated levels of acculturative stress. They found that perceived family dysfunction and nonpositive "expectations for the future" were significant predictors of acculturative stress; and that acculturative stress, perceived family dysfunction, and nonpositive "expectations for the future" were significant predictors of depression and suicidal ideation. Their overall results suggest that some acculturating Latino adolescents experience high levels of acculturative stress, and that these adolescents are also "at risk" for experiencing critical levels of depression and suicidal ideation. Positive family functioning and positive expectations towards the future may act as buffers against acculturative stress.

DEPRESSION AND PSYCHIATRIC SYMPTOMATOLOGY AMONG MEXICAN AMERICANS

As with suicidality, relatively few studies of depression in the Mexican-American population exist and, again, most of these focus on adults. There are, moreover, no consistent findings in this area. In looking at the relationship between acculturation level and depression, for example, some findings (e.g., Salgado de Snyder, 1987; Vega, Kolody, Valle, & Hough, 1986; Vega, Warheit, Buhl-Auth, & Meinhardt, 1984; Vega, Warheit, & Palacio, 1985) suggest that acculturation level is negatively associated to depressive symptoms, whereas other studies find either the opposite connection (e.g., Burnam, Hough, Karno, Escobar, & Telles, 1987; Golding & Burnam, 1990) or no relationship between acculturation and depressive symptoms (e.g., Burnam, Timbers, & Hough, 1984; Griffith, 1983; Moscicki, Locke, Rae, & Boyd, 1989).

Vega et al. (1984) reported findings from an epidemiologic field study conducted among Mexican Americans and Anglos living in Santa Clara, California. The investigators found that females, those with disrupted marriages, those with low educational achievement, and those under 30 years of age had significantly higher levels of depressive symptoms than their counterparts; and that Spanish-speaking Mexican Americans reported significantly higher levels of depressive symptoms than Anglos and English-speaking Mexican Americans.

Given the relatively high prevalence of depressive symptoms reported among Mexican-American women, both Salgado de Snyder (1987) and Vega et al. (1986) explored depressive symptoms and their correlates among immigrant Mexican women. In a sample of married women in Los Angeles County, Salgado de Snyder found significant associations between levels of depressive symptoms and acculturative stress, lack of English proficiency, lack of spousal support, and lack of control over the decision to migrate. Similarly, Vega et al., in a sample of Mexican immigrant women in San Diego County, found significant associations between depressive symptoms and recent migration, low family income, low educational achievement, reduced health status, disrupted marital status, and the lack of confidant support. Both Salgado de Snyder's and Vega et al.'s samples revealed a high prevalence of depression (64% caseness on CES-D and 42% caseness on CES-D, respectively). Their overall findings suggest that a relatively high proportion of Mexican immigrant women may be at risk for the development of psychological problems.

Vega et al. (1985) explored psychiatric symptomatology within a sample of Mexican-American farmworkers in central California and found associations between level of psychiatric symptoms, environmental stressors, and reduced health status. Middle-aged individuals reported elevated symptom levels. The authors conjectured that middle age is an especially high-risk period for farmworkers since significant occupational and life hazards exist to degrade farmworker's health and functional capacities, and farmworkers have few available resources for health maintenance or preventive care. According to Vega et al., the severe lifestyle (high frequencies of environmental stressors, including hazardous working conditions) of Mexican-American farmworkers places them at extraordinary psychiatric risk.

Contrary to the above four studies, the findings of Burnam et al. (1987) and Golding and Burnam (1990) do not suggest a negative association between depressive symptoms and acculturation level. Burnam et al. looked at acculturation and lifetime prevalence of major DSM-III (American Psychiatric Association, 1980) psychiatric disorders among Mexican-American adults in Los Angeles. The authors found that the group of Mexican Americans they defined as "more acculturated" had increased lifetime rates of phobia and substance abuse or dependence; and that United States-born Mexican Americans had a higher prevalence of depressive disorders than did immigrant Mexican Americans. Similarly, Golding and Burnam, in their assessment of depressive symptoms among Mexican Americans in Los Angeles, found that U.S.-born Mexican Americans reported more depressive symptoms than immigrant Mexican Americans. Tests of interaction terms suggested that the U.S.-born Mexican Americans were more vulnerable to the effects of low acculturation than were the immigrant Mexican Americans. According to the authors, this immigrant status difference was possibly due to unmeasured variables such as the selective migration of persons with better coping skills and the selective return of depressed individuals to Mexico.

Only a handful of studies (Emslie, Weinberg, Rush, Adams, & Rintelmann, 1990; Hovey & King, 1996; Roberts & Sobhan, 1992; Swanson et al., 1992; Weinberg & Emslie, 1987) have addressed depression among Mexican-American adolescents. Generally, these studies revealed a high prevalence of depressive symptoms among Mexican-American adolescents in comparison to both Anglo adolescents (Emslie et al., 1990; Roberts & Sobhan, 1992; Weinberg & Emslie, 1987) and Mexican adolescents (Swanson et al., 1992).

FATALISM AND CATHOLICISM

It should be noted that both the concept of fatalism and the Catholic religion have been theorized to affect levels of psychological distress within the Mexican-American population. A long-standing assumption among behavioral scientists (e.g., Edmonson, 1957; Madsen, 1973) is that fatalism (external control) is a prominent characteristic of Mexican-American culture. As stated by Madsen (1973, p. 18), within Mexican-American culture "it is generally believed that the good or bad fortune of the individual is predestined and every occurrence in human existence comes to pass because it was fated to do so." A belief in external control is associated with psychological distress because it reduces both the will and the ability to cope with life's problems (Pearlin, Liebermann, Menaghan, & Mullan, 1981). Other authors (e.g., Casavantes, 1970), however, have argued that fatalism is not a characteristic of Mexican-American culture, but a function of socioeconomic factors. Mexican Americans are fatalistic because they tend to be poor.

Previous research on fatalism among Mexican Americans have revealed inconsistent findings. For example, Buriel and Rivera (1980) found that ethnic differences in locus of control disappeared when they statistically controlled for family income. Their findings lend support to the notion of fatalism as a class-bound characteristic. Chandler (1979), on the other hand, controlled for occupation and education and found that Mexican Americans were more likely than Anglos to believe in external control. Mirowsky and Ross (1984) and Ross, Mirowsky, and Cockerham (1983) controlled for income and found that fatalistic attitudes among Mexican Americans resulted in greater levels of depressive symptoms. They suggested that this relationship is counterbalanced by protective aspects of Mexican-American culture, such as strong levels of family support and social support.

Another long held belief is that the Catholic religion is an inherent part of Mexican-American culture (Mosqueda, 1986). Catholicism may influence suicide among Mexican Americans in a couple of ways. First, the Catholic religion itself may serve as a deterrent against suicide. Within the religion it is considered a sin to take a life under any circumstances, and religious concepts – such as the belief in an afterlife – may make suffering more endurable and thus lower the risk for suicide. Thus, given Catholicism's ideology, those most involved religiously would be expected to reveal less suicide (Maris, 1981; Stack, 1992).

The Catholic religion may further play a protective role through its influence on cultural norms. Within Mexican-American culture, religious ceremonies (e.g., Baptism, Communion, Confirmation, the Quinceañera, the "Day of the Dead" celebration) are considered social events. These celebrations strengthen bonds among family and friends, and extend support systems. As an example, the baptismal ceremony is the foundation for *compadrazgo* (being a Godparent). A *compadre* (Godparent) is expected to accept religious and social obligations to the Godchild and the Godchild's family. These responsibilities are usually accepted even during those instances when compadres do not consider themselves to be religious (Mosqueda, 1986). Thus, oftentimes the responsibilities formed through religious ceremonies such as compadrazgo function primarily as social obligations.

METHODOLOGICAL CONSIDERATIONS

In looking over past research on suicide and risk factors among immigrant and Mexican-American groups, several methodological issues of importance stand out. First of all, as noted earlier, several studies of suicidality within immigrant (e.g., Boor, 1981; Lester, 1989; Stack, 1981a, 1981b; Trovato, 1986a, 1986b) and Mexican-American samples (e.g., Anatore & Loya, 1973; Hatcher & Hatcher, 1975; Hoppe & Martin, 1986; Smith et al., 1985) have focused on suicide rate. These studies have been especially helpful in detailing both the connection between suicide rate and immigrant status, and the elevated suicide rates within specific Mexican-American age groups. At the same time, however, the predominance of such investigations highlights the paucity of research pertinent to the full continuum of suicidal behavior. For example, to our knowledge, only four published studies (Hovey & King, 1996; Sorenson & Golding, 1988a, 1988b; Swanson et al., 1992) have explored suicidal ideation among Mexican Americans. Of these, only Sorenson and Golding (1988a, 1988b) have examined suicide attempts among Mexican Americans. Further exploration of variables that are sometimes precursors to suicide – suicidal ideation and nonlethal attempts – among immigrants and acculturating Mexican Americans is thus imperative, as is the need for precise measurement and statistical analyses of the variables of theoretical interest (e.g., when possible, using regression analyses to explore specific conceptually based research questions).

The second issue of concern relates, to some degree, to the notion of variance within acculturating groups. A large proportion of past research on immigrants, in general, and Mexican-American immigrant–ethnic groups, in specific, either fails to address or ignores variability within groups (see Zuckerman, 1990, for a discussion of the exploration of variance within groups). In the studies that investigated the relationship between immigrant status and suicide rate (e.g., Boor, 1981; Lester, 1989; Stack, 1981a, 1981b; Trovato, 1986a, 1986b), the groups of interest consisted of immigrants of different ethnicities. Such studies, however, are inherently limited. Although these studies are valuable in pointing out the connection between immigrant status and suicide rate, they fail to provide new information about specific ethnic groups. To some extent, the findings of such studies depend on particular sets of immigrants sampled. Lester (1989, p. 1298) appears to recognize this when he states that the replication of findings on the relationship between immigration and suicide rate depends on the "particular sample nations chosen for the analyses." We need to acknowledge that characteristics among particular ethnic groups may vary. Immigrant Irish Americans, for example, may reveal variables of interest that differ from those of immigrant Japanese Americans. Given these concerns, a study such as that reported by Smith et al. (1985), which explores suicide rate within a specific ethnic context, is welcome.

We must also acknowledge variability within particular ethnic populations. For example, several studies have compared the prevalence of suicidality (e.g., Hoppe & Martin, 1986; Sorenson & Golding, 1988a, 1988b; Smith et al., 1985) or symptomatology (e.g., Burnam et al., 1984; Roberts & Sobhan, 1992; Vega et al., 1984) among Mexican Americans and Anglos.

This is useful for epidemiological purposes. Until somewhat recently, we had no information pertaining to the prevalence of depressive and other psychiatric symptomatology among ethnic minority populations (see Vega & Rumbaut, 1991). However, there are major difficulties inherent in any effort to generalize across the entire acculturating Mexican-American population. It is difficult to answer questions such as:

Are Mexican Americans more depressed than Anglos?
Are Mexican Americans more at risk for developing psychiatric disorders?

Some studies suggest yes. Some studies do not. These questions are very general and it is almost impossible to make general statements, given the variance found within the population of acculturating Mexican Americans.

Not all Mexican Americans are suicidal or depressed. It seems likely, for example, that migrant farmworkers living a severe, migratory lifestyle may be more prone to distress than individuals living a more stable, supported (by family and community) lifestyle in Los Angeles. What is important is that we rephrase our questions of interest; for example:

Which Mexican Americans are depressed?
Which Mexican Americans are suicidal?
What are the (immediate) factors that contribute to or buffer suicidality and depression found among Mexican Americans?

Some researchers have begun to explore risk within the Mexican-American population. For example, we have findings that suggest that some immigrant women (e.g., Salgado de Snyder, 1987; Vega et al., 1986), adolescents experiencing high levels of acculturative stress (Hovey & King, 1996), and farmworkers (Vega et al., 1985) may be at extreme risk for the development of psychiatric problems. On the other hand, variables such as (among others) family support (e.g., Hovey & King, 1996; Vega, Kolody, Valle, & Weir, 1991), social support (e.g., Padilla et al., 1988), spousal support (Salgado de Snyder, 1987; Sorenson & Golding, 1988b), positive cognitive attributes (Hovey & King, 1996), and English-language proficiency (Padilla et al., 1988; Salgado de Snyder, 1987; Vega et al., 1985) may help buffer against distress.

This last point closely relates to our third methodological consideration, namely the need to identify and examine the precise aspects of culture that relate to suicidality and depressive and other symptomatology. As mentioned, several "cross-cultural" studies have looked at suicidality and depression among immigrants and Mexican Americans through the use of comparison groups. This type of research, however, does not address the question "What about the culture influences suicidality and depression?" It is one thing to note that a specific cultural group is at risk. It is something else to begin to answer the question of why specific individuals within the group may be at risk. We can begin to answer the question of why by striving to be precise with our research – that is, by being specific with our research questions, our theoretical constructs of interest, our corresponding operational definitions and measures, and the characteristics of populations sampled.

As an example, Betancourt and Lopez (1993) note that several studies – in examining the relationship between level of acculturation and psychological distress – confound the notions of acculturation and acculturative stress in their interpretations of results. Level of acculturation may also indirectly reflect other less general variables such as "adherence to specific cultural values." To better measure specific cultural influences without the possible confounding of variables, researchers should incorporate specific measures of culture-relevant variables (e.g., using an acculturative stress scale if pertinent to the conceptual model).

Finally, past studies of suicidality and depression among immigrant and Mexican-American groups rarely have made use of qualitative methodology. In this literature there is very little, for example, that is reported in respect to open-ended interviews (for an example, see Padilla et al., 1988). Although qualitative methodology, by itself, does not give us the same statistical power as quantitative methods, in conjunction they can be very revealing. Adding qualitative methods – in a research design – to those more quantitative allows for a depth and richness in the data. As a result of the lack of qualitative data in past research, a "sense of the individual," a sense of individual experience, is almost completely missing. Certainly it is rare that we find a quotation such as the one that begins this article.

EXAMPLE OF QUALITATIVE METHODOLOGY

Let us briefly turn our attention back to Hovey and King (1996). As noted earlier, in a sample of immigrant and second-generation Latino-American (87% Mexican American) adolescents, we examined the relationship between acculturative stress, depressive symptoms, and suicidal ideation; and determined the best predictors of elevated levels of acculturative stress, depression, and suicidal ideation. For this particular study, our research design was guided by the model of acculturative stress, depression, and suicidal ideation (see Fig. 1) that we presented earlier. Using multiple regression analyses, we found that there were significant relationships between acculturative stress, depression, and suicidal ideation; that perceived family dysfunction and nonpositive "expectations toward the future" were significant predictors of acculturative stress; and that acculturative stress, perceived family dysfunction, and nonpositive expectations toward the future were significant predictors of depression and suicidal ideation. Thus, within this sample, it appears that those acculturating individuals experiencing heightened levels of acculturative stress are "at risk" for experiencing critical levels of depression and suicidal ideation, and that family support and positive expectations toward the future may moderate (buffer against) levels of distress (for a more thorough discussion of these findings, we refer the reader to Hovey & King, 1996). It is our belief that the acculturative stress model holds promise for future research of depression and suicidal ideation among acculturating groups.

In designing that study (Hovey & King, 1996) we were also guided by the methodological concerns discussed in the present paper. For example, to help ascertain which acculturating adolescents are at risk, we explored within-group differences; and in comparison to previous studies of depression and suicidal ideation among acculturating Mexican Americans, we used acculturative stress (focusing on degree of difficulty experienced by acculturating individuals) as our "starting point," rather than level of acculturation. In addition, to further gather an experiential sense of the acculturating adolescents, we collected qualitative data. In measuring expectations toward the future, we asked, "What do you think the future will be like for you and your family?" We coded each response as positive (hopeful), neutral, or nonpositive (nonhopeful).

An underlying theme of the present paper has been that of "not losing a sense of the individual." In keeping with this theme, we would like to take this opportunity to share some of the adolescents' responses to the question concerning their future. These responses are revealing in that they deliver a sense of richness, immediacy, and individual experience not found in mere numbers.

The first response is from a 17-year-old female and points to the possible links among future expectations, family support, and acculturative stress:

> Well, I hope and trust in God that my family's future will be better. I hope that I will become something in life and that my family will be proud of me. I hope that we will all understand each other better and that everyone's dreams will be realized.

These next responses reveal the desire for, and the notion that hard work can lead to happiness and success:

> I think that only by moving forward can our future be good; not a success but not one of sadness either. I think that it will go well if we set our minds to it, and always forge ahead with much effort. (15-year-old female)

> Well, I think it can be a good future, because I'll be able to graduate and study a career that will help me triumph [succeed] in the future. All in my family plan to better ourselves for our own well-being. (16-year-old female)

> I will study until I learn English and graduate; to have a good job and be able to help my family in the future; and not to have more problems between my family and me. (16-year-old male)

> My future depends on how I live now but I think that if we all continue to work as we have, our future will be good. Although I would like to have my own family, I would like for my family's plans and goals to become a reality; one of these is to live happily and financially well off as a good and happy family. That is all that I think can be done in order to have a good happy future. (19-year-old female)

These last two responses are from adolescents who reveal nonhopeful outlooks toward their future. The first is from an 18-year-old female, briefly expressing her outlook in a blunt manner. The second is from a 17-year-old male who reveals sarcasm in expressing his dissatisfaction with his current life situation:

> It will be depressing.

> I'm going to go to Mexico to live with my father. My mother is going to be rich and old.

CONCLUSION

The immigrant population in the United States has increased dramatically over the past two decades. This increase is best represented through statistics, which are compelling. Nearly half of the immigrant population in the United States (21.2 million as of 1990) has entered the country since 1980 (Passel & Edmonston, 1992). About one fourth of the nation's immigrant population arrive in California (approximately 250,000 each year) (Stewart, 1993). According to the 1990 census figures (U.S. Department of Commerce, 1993), Latino individuals in California number more than 7.5 million (one fourth of the state's population). Of these individuals, 45% are immigrants, and 85% of these immigrants are of Mexican origin. These statistics do not take into account the undocumented and the uncounted.

Our current knowledge of suicidality among Mexican Americans is limited. However, there is evidence that suggests that some acculturating Mexican Americans may be at an increased risk for suicide. Mexican Americans in the southwest United States have revealed (Smith et al., 1985) an elevated overall suicide rate (9.0 for the period 1976–1980) in comparison to the overall suicide rate found in Mexico (0.7 in 1973) (World Health Organization, 1973). Suicide rates for Mexican Americans decline with age and thus suggest that suicide among Mexican Americans is more of a youthful phenomena. Mexican-American adults born in the United States have revealed (Sorenson & Golding, 1988a) elevated lifetime rates of suicide attempts (4.8% vs. 1.6%) and suicidal ideation (13.0% vs. 4.5%) in comparison to Mexican-American adults born in Mexico. Mexican-American adolescents have revealed (Hovey & King, 1996; Swanson et al., 1992) extremely high levels of suicidal ideation, especially in comparison to Mexican adolescents. Finally, among Mexican-American adolescents, heightened levels of acculturative stress may result in critical levels of suicidal ideation (Hovey & King, 1996). Overall, these findings suggest that acculturating Mexican Americans may feel caught between the influence of traditional values and norms and their experiences in the mainstream society.

As the statistics suggest, the Latino population (comprised predominantly of Mexican Americans) is projected (Portes & Rumbaut, 1990) to become the largest ethnic minority group in the United States by early in the next century. What is striking is that the research this paper addresses pales in comparison to these statistics. It is crucial, in other words, that future research "keeps up" with immigration rates and fully explores depression, suicidal thoughts and behaviors, and completed suicide among immigrant and specific acculturating groups. This paper has reviewed past research of suicidality and depression among immigrant and Mexican-American groups, identified methodological issues of concern, and suggested directions for future research.

Our suggestions for future research of suicide and risk factors among acculturating groups are summarized as follows:

- Further exploration of the continuum of suicidal thoughts and behavior
- Further exploration of the variance within the acculturating population
- Identification and examination of the precise aspects of culture that relate to suicide risk factors
- Research designs that combine quantitative and qualitative methods, to help gain a sense of individual experience

The importance of future research that explores suicidality and symptomatology in a precise manner cannot be understated. It is only through specificity—in the exploration of within-group risk—that research findings can become more applied and thus benefit immigrant-ethnic groups in this country.

REFERENCES

American Psychiatric Association. (1980). *Diagnostic and statistical manual of mental disorders* (3rd ed.). Washington, DC: Author.

Anatore, B., & Loya, F. (1973). *An analysis of minority and white suicide rates in Denver.* Paper presented at the Rocky Mountain Psychological Association, Las Vegas, NV.

Berry, J. W., & Kim, U. (1988). Acculturation and mental health. In P. Dasen, J. W. Berry, & N. Sartorius (Eds.), *Health and cross-cultural psychology: Towards application* (pp. 207-236). London: Sage.

Betancourt, H., & Lopez, S. R. (1993). The study of culture, ethnicity, and race in American psychology. *American Psychologist, 48,* 629-637.

Boor, M. (1981). Relationship of 1977 state suicide rates to population increases and immigration. *Psychological Reports, 49,* 856-858.

Buriel, R., & Rivera, L. (1980). The relationship of locus of control to family income and familism among Anglo- and Mexican-American high school students. *Journal of Social Psychology, 111,* 27-34.

Burnam, M. A., Timbers, D. M., & Hough, R. L. (1984). Two measures of psychological distress among Mexican Americans, Mexicans, and Anglos. *Journal of Health and Social Behavior, 25,* 24-33.

Burnam, M. A., Hough, R. L., Karno, M., Escobar, J. I., & Telles, C. A. (1987). Acculturation and lifetime prevalence of psychiatric disorders among Mexican Americans in Los Angeles. *Journal of Health and Social Behavior, 28,* 89-102.

Casavantes, E. (1970). Pride and prejudice: A Mexican-American dilemma. *Civil Rights Digest, 3,* 22-27.

Chandler, C. R. (1979). Traditionalism in a modern setting: A comparison of Anglo- and Mexican-American value orientations. *Human Organization, 38,* 153-159.

Durkheim, E. (1951). *Suicide.* (J. A. Spaulding & A. G. Simpson, Trans.). New York: Free Press. (Original work published 1897)

Edmonson, M. S. (1957). *Los Manitos: A study of institutional values.* New Orleans: Tulane University Press.

Emslie, G. J., Weinberg, W. A., Rush, A. J., Adams, R. M., & Rintelmann, J. W. (1990). Depressive symptoms by self-report in adolescence: Phase I of the development of a questionnaire for depression by self-report. *Journal of Child Neurology, 5,* 114-121.

Golding, J. M., & Burnam, M. A. (1990). Immigration, stress, and depressive symptoms in a Mexican-American community. *Journal of Nervous and Mental Disease, 178,* 161-171.

Griffith, J. (1983). Relationship between acculturation and psychological impairment in adult Mexican-Americans. *Hispanic Journal of Behavioral Sciences, 5,* 431-459.

Hatcher, C., & Hatcher, D. (1975). Ethnic group suicide: An analysis of Mexican American and Anglo suicide rates for El Paso, Texas. *Crisis Intervention, 6,* 2-9.

Hoppe, S. K., & Martin, H. W. (1986). Patterns of suicide among Mexican-Americans and Anglos, 1960-1980. *Social Psychiatry, 21,* 83-88.

Hovey, J. D., & King, C. A. (1996). Acculturative stress, depression, and suicidal ideation among immigrant and second generation Latino adolescents. *Journal of the American Academy of Child and Adolescent Psychiatry, 35,* 1183-1192.

Lester, D. (1989). Immigration and rates of personal violence (suicide and homicide). *Psychological Reports, 65,* 1298.

Loya, F. (1976). *Increases in Chicano suicide, Denver, Colorado, 1960-1975: What can be done?* Paper presented at the American Association of Suicidology, Los Angeles.

Madsen, W. (1973). *The Mexican-Americans of South Texas* (2nd ed). New York: Holt, Rinehart, & Winston.

Maris, R. M. (1981). *Pathways to suicide: A survey of self-destructive behaviors.* Baltimore: Johns Hopkins University Press.

Mirowsky, J., & Ross, C. E. (1984). Mexican culture and its emotional contradictions. *Journal of Health and Social Behavior, 25,* 2-13.

Moscicki, E., Locke, B., Rae, D., & Boyd, J. (1989). Depressive symptoms among Mexican Americans: The Hispanic Health and Nutrition Examination Survey. *American Journal of Epidemiology, 130,* 348-360.

Mosqueda, L. J. (1986). *Chicanos, Catholicism and*

political ideology. Lanham, MD: University Press of America.

Padilla, A. M., Cervantes, R. C., Maldonado, M., & Garcia, R. E. (1988). Coping responses to psychosocial stressors among Mexican and Central American immigrants. *Journal of Community Psychology, 16,* 418-427.

Passel, J. S., & Edmonston, B. (1992). *Immigration and race in the United States: The 20th and 21st centuries.* Washington, DC: The Urban Institute.

Pearlin, L. I., Lieberman, M. A., Menaghan, E. G., & Mullan, J. T. (1981). The stress process. *Journal of Health and Social Behavior, 22,* 337-356.

Portes, A., & Rumbaut, R. G. (1990). *Immigrant America: A portrait.* Berkeley: University of California Press.

Roberts, R. E., & Sobhan, M. (1992). Symptoms of depression in adolescence: A comparison of Anglo, African, Hispanic Americans. *Journal of Youth and Adolescence, 21,* 639-651.

Ross, C. E., Mirowsky, J. & Cockerham, W. C. (1983). Social class, Mexican culture, and fatalism: Their effects on psychological distress. *American Journal of Community Psychology, 11,* 383-399.

Salgado de Snyder, V. N. (1987). Factors associated with acculturative stress and depressive symptomatology among married Mexican immigrant women. *Psychology of Women Quarterly, 11,* 475-488.

Smith, J. C., Mercy, J. A., & Warren, C. W. (1985). Comparison of suicides among Anglos and Hispanics in five southwestern states. *Suicide and Life-Threatening Behavior, 15,* 14-26.

Sorenson, S. B., & Golding, J. M. (1988a). Prevalence of suicide attempts in a Mexican-American population: Prevention implications of immigration and cultural issues. *Suicide and Life-Threatening Behavior, 18,* 322-333.

Sorenson, S. B., & Golding, J. M. (1988b). Suicide ideation and attempts in Hispanics and non-Hispanic Whites: Demographic and psychiatric disorder issues. *Suicide and Life-Threatening Behavior, 18,* 205-218.

Stack, S. (1981a). Comparative analysis of immigration and suicide. *Psychological Reports, 49,* 509-510.

Stack, S. (1981b). The effect of immigration on suicide: A cross-national analysis. *Basic and Applied Social Psychology, 2,* 205-218.

Stack, S. (1992). Marriage, family, religion, and suicide. In R. W. Maris, A. L. Berman, J. T. Maltsberger, & R. I. Yufit (Eds.), *Assessment and prediction of suicide* (pp. 540-552). New York: Guilford Press.

Stewart, D. W. (1993). *Immigration and education: The crisis and the opportunities.* New York: Lexington Books.

Swanson, J. W., Linskey, A. O., Quintero-Salinas, R., Pumariega, A. J., & Holzer, C. E. (1992). A binational school survey of depressive symptoms, drug use, and suicidal ideation. *Journal of the American Academy of Child and Adolescent Psychiatry, 31,* 669-678.

Trovato, F. (1986a). Suicide and ethnic factors in Canada. *International Journal of Social Psychiatry, 32*(3), 55-64.

Trovato, F. (1986b). A time series analysis of international immigration and suicide mortality in Canada. *International Journal of Social Psychiatry, 32*(2), 38-46.

U.S. Department of Commerce. (1993). *1990 census of population: Social and economic characteristics of California.* Washington, DC: U.S. Department of Commerce.

Vega, W. A., Kolody, B., Valle, R., & Hough, R. (1986). Depressive symptoms and their correlates among immigrant Mexican women in the United States. *Social Science and Medicine, 22,* 645-652.

Vega, W. A., Kolody, B., Valle, R., and Weir, J. (1991). Social networks, social support, and their relationship to depression among immigrant Mexican women. *Human Organization, 50,* 154-162.

Vega, W. A., & Rumbaut, R. G. (1991). Ethnic minorities and mental health. *Annual Review of Sociology, 17,* 351-383.

Vega, W. A., Warheit, G., Buhl-Auth, J., & Meinhardt, K. (1984). The prevalence of depressive symptoms among Mexican Americans and Anglos. *American Journal of Epidemiology, 120,* 592-607.

Vega, W. A., Warheit, G., & Palacio, R. (1985). Psychiatric symptomatology among Mexican American farmworkers. *Social Science and Medicine, 20,* 39-45.

Weinberg, W. A., & Emslie, G. J. (1987). Depression and suicide in adolescents. *International Pediatrics, 2,* 154-159.

Williams, C. L., & Berry, J. W. (1991). Primary prevention of acculturative stress among refugees: Application of psychological theory and practice. *American Psychologist, 46,* 632-641.

World Health Organization (1973). Vital statistics and cause of death. In *World health statistics annual.* Geneva: Author.

Zuckerman, M. (1990). Some dubious premises in research and theory on racial differences: Scientific, social, and ethical issues. *American Psychologist, 45,* 1297-1303.

PART III. International Perspectives

11
Suicide in an International Perspective

David Lester

Epidemiological trends in national suicide rates were identified, including a slowdown in the 1980s in the suicide rates of nations with the highest rates and a rising male suicide rate worldwide. A review of theories of national differences in suicide rates permitted selection of a small set of predictor variables, which were quite successful in predicting the suicide rates of 17 industrialized nations.

One of the most interesting phenomena in suicidology is the national variation in suicide rates. Suicide rates vary tremendously, from a high presently in Hungary and Sri Lanka to a low in Egypt and Kuwait (see Table 1). The differences in national suicides are large and stable. For example, Lester (1987b) found a correlation of 0.42 between the suicide rates of 14 European nations in 1875 and in 1975 – a span of 100 years. Although many doubts have been expressed about the validity of official suicide rates (e.g., Douglas, 1967), Sainsbury and Barraclough (1968) and Lester (1972) have found that the suicide rates of immigrant groups to the United States and to Australia are strongly associated with the suicide rates in the home nations from which they came. Thus, for example, the Irish have a relatively low suicide rate and Irish immigrants to the United States and to Australia, where they encounter the same medical examiners as other immigrant groups, also have relatively low suicide rates. Thus, national suicide rates appear to have some degree of validity.

The goals of the present paper are to present some simple epidemiological facts and trends in national suicide rates, and then to briefly review and illustrate possible explanations for these phenomena.

THE EPIDEMIOLOGY OF SUICIDE WORLDWIDE

The suicide rates of nations around the world circa 1990 are shown in Table 1. What is noteworthy about this table is the number of nations that do not report their mortality statistics to the World Health Organization, especially nations in Africa, the Middle East and Central and South America. As a result, our knowledge of worldwide trends in suicide is limited to the nations that do report their mortality rates.

In all but one of the nations in Table 1, the male suicide rate is higher than the female suicide rate, though the difference is lower in Asian nations than elsewhere; the lone exception is China, where women have a higher suicide rate than men (33.5 per 100,000 per year vs. 24.2 for 1990–1994 – Phillips & Liu, 1996). Lester (1990) found that 21 of 23 nations experienced an increase in the male suicide rate from 1970 to 1984, whereas only 14 of the 23 nations did for the female suicide rate. Thus, while male suicide rates seem to be rising worldwide, female rates do not.

Lester (1988a) found that nations with higher suicide rates in 1970 experienced a larger absolute increase from 1970 to 1980, and he predicted that suicide rates

David Lester is with the Center for the Study of Suicide. Address correspondence to the author at RR 41, 5 Stonegate Court, Blackwood, NJ 08012.

Suicide and Life-Threatening Behavior, Vol. 27(1), Spring 1997

TABLE 1
Suicide Rates Around the World in 1990
(from the World Health Organization Unless Otherwise Noted)

Nation	Rate	Comment
Hungary	39.9	
Sri Lanka	33.2	(1900 rates not available) 1986 data
Finland	30.3	
China	28.7	(Phillips & Liu, 1996) 1990–1994
Slovenia	27.6	
Estonia	27.1	
Russian Federation	26.5	
Lithuania	26.1	
Latvia	26.0	
Germany, East	24.4	
Denmark	24.1	
Austria	23.6	
Belarus	23.6	(1990 rates not available) 1992 data
Switzerland	21.9	
USSR	21.1	
Ukraine	20.7	
Byelorussia	20.4	
France	20.1	
Belgium	19.3	(1990 rates not available) 1989 data
Czech Republic	19.3	
Kazakhstan	19.1	
Czechoslovakia	17.9	
Luxembourg	17.8	
Germany, West	17.5	
Germany	17.5	(1990 rates not available) 1991 data
Sweden	17.2	
Japan	16.4	
Iceland	15.7	
Norway	15.5	
Yugoslavia	15.3	
Bulgaria	14.7	
Mauritius	14.2	
Trinidad & Tobago	13.7	
New Zealand	13.5	
Singapore	13.1	
Poland	13.0	
Australia	12.9	
Canada	12.7	
Kyrgyzstan	12.5	
USA	12.4	
Hong Kong	11.7	
Puerto Rico	10.5	
Scotland	10.5	
Uruguay	10.3	
Northern Ireland	9.9	
Netherlands	9.7	
Ireland	9.5	
Romania	9.0	
Portugal	8.8	
United Kingdom	8.1	
Korea, South	8.0	(1990 rates not available) 1987 data
England & Wales	7.8	
Italy	7.6	
Spain	7.5	
Zimbabwe	7.4	(Mugadza, 1996)
Uzbekistan	6.8	(1990 rates not available) 1991 data

(*continued*)

TABLE 1
Continued

Nation	Rate	Comment
Liechtenstein	6.7	
Argentina	6.7	
Taiwan	6.7	(Andrew Cheng)
Israel	6.5	
Chile	5.6	(1990 rates not available) 1989 data
Costa Rica	5.2	
Venezuela	4.8	(1990 rates not available) 1989 data
Barbados	4.7	(1990 rates not available) 1988 data
Ecuador	4.6	(1990 rates not available) 1988 data
Macao	4.4	(1990 rates not available) 1987 data
Panama	3.8	(1990 rates not available) 1987 data
Tadjikistan	3.8	(1990 rates not available) 1991 data
Greece	3.5	
Bahrain	3.1	(1990 rates not available) 1988 data
Colombia	3.1	(1990 rates not available) 1991 data
Armenia	2.8	
Malta	2.3	
Mexico	2.3	
St Lucia	2.3	(1990 rates not available) 1987 data
Albania	2.1	(1990 rates not available) 1989 data
Maldives	2.0	(1990 rates not available) 1987 data
Bahamas	1.2	(1990 rates not available) 1987 data
Kuwait	0.8	(1990 rates not available) 1987 data
Egypt	0.04	(1990 rates not available) 1987 data

would continue to rise worldwide. However, Lester (1995) found that the nations with the lower suicide rates in 1980 experienced the larger increase during the 1980s, opposite to his finding for the 1970s.

Lester (1982) found that the male suicide rate rose with age in most nations of the world. For females, the distribution of suicide rates by age varied with the level of economic development of the nation. For the wealthiest nations, female suicide rates tended to peak in middle age. For poorer nations, the peak shifted to elderly women, whereas for the poorest nations, the peak shifted to young adult women. More recently, Girard (1993) confirmed that the distribution of suicide rates by age depended upon the level of economic development of the nation

In the 1970s there was concern over both rising elderly suicide rates (Lester, 1993) and rising youth suicide rates (Lester 1988b). Data for the 1980s are shown in Table 2, where it can be seen that nations were equally likely to experience an increase or a decrease in male overall suicide rates, in male youth and male elderly suicide rates, and in female elderly suicide rates. The majority of nations experienced a decrease in female overall suicide rates and in female youth suicide rates.

Using time-series multiple regression analyses, Lester (1994b) found that suicide rates in nations of the world from 1950 to 1985 were significantly associated with higher divorce rates and lower birth and marriage rates in the majority of the 21 nations studied, as predicted by Durkheim's (1897) classic theory of suicide.

PREDICTING NATIONAL SUICIDE RATES

A number of studies have appeared in recent years examining social correlates of national suicide rates. It is of interest to inquire, therefore, whether the results of this research could be used to identify a

TABLE 2
Percentage Change in Youth and Elderly Suicide Rates from 1980 to 1990

	Change (%)					
	Males			Females		
	Total	Youth	Elderly	Total	Youth	Elderly
Australia	+26	+51	−2	−7	+4	−13
Austria	−8	−13	+26	−10	−18	+5
Bulgaria	+8	+25	−11	+7	−43	+22
Canada	−4	−1	−15	−24	−7	−29
Costa Rica	−45	−6	+14	+14	−65	+infinity
Czechoslovakia	−10	−38	−5	−10	−4	−10[a]
Denmark	−12	−13	−6	−27	−87	+2
England & Wales	+10	+83	−10	−45	−33	−44
Finland	+19	+36	+50	+16	+21	+5
France	+6	−10	+6	0	−19	+5
Greece	+17	+73	+5	−21	+83	−61
Hong Kong	−12	−10	+6	−14	−12	−29
Hungary	−7	−36	−3	−19	+2	−17
Ireland	+73	+154	+289	+9	+21	−47
Israel	+17	−38	−1	−5	+175	−47
Italy	+13	+11	+34	−11	−17	−8
Japan	−8	−45	−14	−5	−43	−19
Netherlands	−4	−1	−17	−3	−3	+24
New Zealand	+51	+95	+8	−24	−17	−65
N. Ireland	+107	+87	+20	+56	+213	+61
Norway	+27	+8	+29	+21	+91	+68
Portugal	+21	+42	+8	+15	−24	+45
Puerto Rico	+24	−19	+39	−25	−24	−100
Scotland	+30	+72	−7	−37	−42	−60
Singapore	+19	+48	−26	+15	−34	+14
Spain	+67	+65	+81	+86	+55	+102
Sweden	−13	−13	+13	−8	−9	+31
Switzerland	−14	−27	+8	−16	−49	+1
United States	+10	+9	+33	−11	−9	+11
USSR	−24	−24	+6	−16	+5	+6
West Germany	−21	−21	−1	−32	−20	−8
Yugoslavia	+4	−5	+22	+6	−36	+28

[a]The data for Czechoslovakia are for 1981 to 1990 since 1980 data were not published by the World Health Organization.

set of social variables that can predict national suicide rates.

Physiological Theories

One possible explanation, of course, for differences in the suicide rates of nations is that different nationalities differ in some relevant manner in their physiology. Perhaps, for example, there are differences in inherited psychiatric disorders, particularly affective disorders, or in brain concentrations of serotonin, the neurotransmitter believed to be responsible for depression. As yet, there are no data to test these possibilities for a large sample of nations. However, Lester (1991) found that estimated β_{max} levels of ^{3}H-imipramine platelet binding sites (a possible biochemical indicator of endogenous depressive disorder) in members of eight nations were significantly associated with the suicide rates of those nations. Thus, future research may identify physiological correlates of national suicide rates in a large sample of nations.

Lester (1987a) studied the associations between the proportions of people in 17 industrialized nations with the different types of blood (O, A, B, and AB) and the nations' suicide rates. He found that, the lower the proportion of Type O people and the higher the proportion of Type AB people, the higher the suicide rate.

Mawson and Jacobs (1978) noted that the synthesis of the neurotransmitter serotonin (believed to contribute to people's level of depression) by the body requires the precursor amino acid L-tryptophan. Corn has less L-tryptophan as compared to other cereals, and so nations with a higher corn consumption would get less L-tryptophan, and so might have lower levels of serotonin. Lester (1985), however, in a study of 38 nations, found no association between per capita consumption of corn and suicide rates. Kitahara (1986a, 1986b) estimated the levels of tryptophan in the blood relative to other amino acids (such as tyrosine) from dietary intake in residents of nations. He found no associations in a large sample of nations (a result replicated by Lester, 1989).

Psychological Theories

The major psychological factors found to be associated with and predictive of suicidal behavior are depression (in particular, hopelessness) and psychological disturbance, labeled variously as neuroticism, anxiety, or emotional instability (Lester, 1992a). Psychiatric disorder of any kind appears to increase the risk of suicide, with affective disorders and substance abuse leading the list.

Alcohol abuse and drug abuse are strongly linked with suicidal behavior. Not only are these behaviors seen as self-destructive in themselves (Menninger, 1938 called them *chronic suicide*), but both attempted and completed suicide occur at high rates in substance abusers (Lester, 1992b).

Composition Theories

Moksony (1990) has noted that one simple explanation of differences in suicide rates between nations is that the national populations differ in the proportion of those at risk for suicide. For example, typically in developed nations, suicide rates are highest in the elderly. Therefore, nations with a higher proportion of the elderly will have a higher suicide rate.

Social Theories

The most popular explanations of social suicide rates focus on social variables. These social variables may be viewed in two ways: (1) as direct causal agents of the suicidal behavior, or (2) as indices of broader, more abstract, social characteristics that differ between nations.

The most important theory for choosing relevant variables is that of Durkheim (1897). Durkheim hypothesized that the societal suicide rate was determined by the society's level of social integration (i.e., the degree to which the people are bound together in social networks) and the level of social regulation (i.e., the degree to which people's desires and emotions are regulated by societal norms and customs). Durkheim thought that this association was curvilinear, but later sociologists have suggested that the association is linear in modern societies (Johnson, 1965), with suicide increasing as social integration and regulation decrease. Studies of samples of nations have found that suicide rates are associated with such variables as the birth rate, female participation in the labor force, immigration, and the divorce rate (Stack, 1980, 1981a, 1981b). Some investigators see these associations as suggesting a direct link between, say, divorce or immigration and suicidal behavior. For example, divorce may be associated with suicide at the aggregate level because divorced people have a higher suicide rate than those with other marital statuses. Other investigators see the associations as suggesting that divorce and immigration are measures of a broader and more basic social characteristic, perhaps social integration, which plays a causal role in suicide. In this latter case, nations with a higher rate of divorce may have a higher rate of suicide for those in all marital statuses.

In a cross-sectional (ecological) study of 25 nations in 1970, Lester (1994a) found that suicide rates were associated positively with the percentage of the elderly, the divorce rate, and the gross domestic product; and negatively with the percentage of people under the age of 15, the unemployment rate, and the birth rate. The association of suicide with birth and divorce rates is consistent with predictions from Durkheim's theory, the association with the percentage of elderly and young is consistent with a composition explanation of the suicide rate, and the association with unemployment and gross domestic product is consistent with previous research findings (Platt, 1984; Stack 1981b).

Predicting Rates

This brief review of physiological, psychological, sociological and compositional theories of suicide rates has identified a number of variables that ought theoretically to be associated with suicide rates or that have been found empirically to correlate with suicide rates. As a test of the utility of these variables, a set of these variables was tested for their ability to predict the suicide rates of a sample of developed nations with available data.

The variables chosen, together with their theoretical source, were: blood type (physiological), alcohol consumption (psychological), percentage of the elderly (compositional), and divorce and birth rates (sociological). The sample used consisted of 18 industrialized nations first used by Lynn (1982) in a study of national character. Data on blood types were available for 17 of these, and the multiple linear regression equation was derived from these 17 nations. The results of the multiple regression analysis are shown in Table 3, where the five predictor variables can be seen to have provided a multiple R of 0.69.

TABLE 3
Results of the Multiple Regression Analysis Predicting the Suicide Rate in 17 Industrialized Nations

	Beta coefficient
Birth rate	−0.07
Divorce rate	0.12
Alcohol consumption	0.26
% elderly	0.17
Blood type	−0.48
R	0.69

Multivariate Analyses

Although there have been studies that have examined the associations between suicide rates and a small number of social variables, only two studies have examined the associations between a large set of social variables and national suicides, both using factor analysis.

Conklin and Simpson (1987) identified two clusters of variables that were associated with national suicide rates: one cluster had the highest loading from the Islam religion and the second cluster seemed to assess economic development. Suicide rates were lower in nations with less economic development and where Islam was a more important religion. Two other clusters (Christianity and the Eastern bloc) were not associated with suicide rates.

Lester (1996), in a similar study of the social correlates of national suicide rates, identified 13 orthogonal (independent) factors for the social variables, only one of which was associated with suicide rates; this factor seemed to measure economic development (with high loadings from such social variables as low population growth and high gross domestic product per capita). Thus, these two studies agreed in finding that economic development is associated with higher suicide rates.

DISCUSSION

Whereas in the 1970s, worldwide suicide rates appeared to be rising, the 1980s witnessed a leveling off of the suicide rates in nations with the highest suicide rates. On the other hand, in the 1980s, nations with relatively lower suicide rates experienced a growth in their suicide rates, which may reflect in part more accurate counting and reporting of suicide in those nations, in addition to socioeconomic changes that may have increased the societal rate of suicide.

The suicide rate of women appears to have decreased in recent years, and the distribution of suicide rates by age appears to have shifted, with youth suicide rates now much higher than they were 20 years ago.

Although theories have been proposed to account for the differences in national suicide rates, these competing theories have not been compared for their usefulness in predicting national suicide rates. In the present paper, a small set of variables drawn from the competing theories proved moderately successful in predicting the suicide rates of 17 nations. However, data are not presently available to carry out such a test on a larger sample of nations.

Finally, it is noteworthy that many nations do not presently report mortality rates in general, and suicide rates in particular, to the World Health Organization. Data from Central and South America, Africa, and the Middle East were conspicuously absent. Thus, our knowledge of worldwide trends in suicide is biased. It is to be hoped that the reporting and investigation of suicide will become more widespread in the world in the 21st century.

REFERENCES

Conklin, G. H., & Simpson, M. E. (1987). The family, socioeconomic development and suicide. *Journal of Comparative Family Studies, 18*, 99–111.

Douglas, J. D. (1967). *The social meanings of suicide.* Princeton: Princeton University.

Durkheim, E. (1897). *Le suicide.* Paris: Felix Alcan.

Girard, C. (1993). Age, gender, and suicide. *American Sociological Review, 58*, 553–574.

Johnson, B. D. (1965). Durkheim's one cause of suicide. *American Sociological Review, 30*, 875–886.

Kitahara, M. (1986a). Dietary tryptophan ratio and suicide. *International Journal of Biosocial Research, 8*(1), 53–60.

Kitahara, M. (1986b). Tryptophan uptake from diet and the incidence of suicide. *Biology & Society, 3*(2), 74–79.

Lester, D. (1972). Migration and suicide. *Medical Journal of Australia, i*, 941–942.

Lester, D. (1982). The distribution of sex and age among completed suicides. *International Journal of Social Psychiatry, 28*, 256–260.

Lester, D. (1985). Corn consumption, tryptophan and cross-national homicide and suicide rates. *Journal of Orthomolecular Psychiatry, 14*, 178–179.

Lester, D. (1987a). National distribution of blood groups, personal violence (suicide and homicide), and national character. *Personality & Individual Differences, 8*, 575–576.

Lester, D. (1987b). The stability of national suicide rates in Europe. *Sociology & Social Research, 71*, 208.

Lester, D. (1988a). A critical-mass theory of national suicide rates. *Suicide & Life-Threatening Behavior, 18*, 279–284.

Lester, D. (1988b). Youth suicide. *Adolescence, 23*, 955–958.

Lester, D. (1989). Tryptophan uptake and national rates of suicide and homicide. *Journal of Orthomolecular Medicine, 4*, 159–160.

Lester, D. (1990). Changes to suicide rates unique to Canada? *Canadian Journal of Public Health, 81*, 240–241.

Lester, D. (1991). The association between platelet imipramine binding sites and suicide. *Pharmacopsychiatry, 24*, 232.

Lester, D. (1992a). *Why people kill themselves.* Springfield, IL: C. C. Thomas.

Lester, D. (1992b). Alcoholism and drug abuse. In R. W. Maris, A. L. Berman, J. T. Maltsberger, & R. I. Yufit (Eds.), *Assessment and prediction of suicide* (pp. 321–336). New York: Guilford Press.

Lester, D. (1993). Attempts to explain changing elderly suicide rates. *International Journal of Geriatric Psychiatry, 8* 435–437.

Lester, D. (1994a). *Patterns of suicide and homicide around the world.* Commack, NY: Nova Science.

Lester, D. (1994b). Domestic integration and suicide in 21 nations, 1950–1985. *International Journal of Comparative Sociology, 35*, 132–137.

Lester, D. (1995). Changes in national suicide rates, 1980–1990. *Psychological Reports, 77*, 906.

Lester, D. (1996). *Suicide and homicide around the world.* Commack, NY: Nova Science.

Lynn, R. (1982). National differences in anxiety and extraversion. *Progress in Experimental Personality Research, 11*, 213–258.

Mawson, A., & Jacobs, K. (1978). Corn consumption, tryptophan and cross-national homicide rates. *Journal of Orthomolecular Psychiatry, 7*, 227–230.

Menninger, K. (1938). *Man against himself.* New York: Harcourt, Brace & World.

Moksony, F. (1990). Ecological analysis of suicide. In D. Lester (Ed.), *Current concepts of suicide* (pp. 121–138). Philadelphia: Charles Press.

Mugadza, W. (July, 1996). *Suicide attempts among young callers in Zimbabwe.* Paper presented at the Befrienders Conference, Kuala Lumpur, Malaysia.

Phillips, M. R., & Liu, H. Q. (July, 1996). *Suicide in China.* Paper presented at the Befrienders Conference, Kuala Lumpur, Malaysia.

Platt, S. (1984). Unemployment and suicidal behavior. *Social Science & Medicine, 19*, 93–115.

Sainsbury, P., & Barraclough, B. M. (1968). Differences between suicide rates. *Nature, 220*, 1252.

Stack, S. (1980). Domestic integration and the rate of suicide. *Journal of Comparative Family Studies, 11*, 249-260.

Stack, S. (1981a). The effect of immigration on suicide. *Basic & Applied Social Psychology, 2*, 205–218.

Stack, S. (1981b). Suicide and religion. *Sociological Focus, 14*, 207–220.

12
Suicide in Canada with Special Reference to the Difference Between Canada and the United States

Isaac Sakinofsky, MD, and Antoon A. Leenaars, PhD

The report of Canada's National Task Force on Suicide (Expert Working Group, 1994) begins: "Suicide . . . eventually, in one way or another, touches the lives of most Canadians." Despite this, systematic suicide data collection began only in 1924, encompassing the whole country since 1956. The pattern of its suicide rates resembles that of the United States but during the 1970s, and for over a decade, Canadian rates in several age categories, particularly males 15–34, overtook them (Leenaars & Lester, 1994; Sakinofsky & Roberts, 1987). Though not far apart, the differences underline the similarities and variations between these neighboring societies (Leenaars, 1995). In this paper we review studies of suicide in Canada and examine the relatedness between suicide phenomena in these two nations.

At the beginning of the Great Depression suicide rates in males in Canada rose and then fell during World War II, but rates in women cycled at a low amplitude close to baseline (Fig. 1). Presumably, these secular changes expressed societal pressures on specific sectors. Until the end of World War II suicide rates in youths of both genders aged 10–19 remained low, as if sheltered from the turbulent social events of the day. After the war, rates in young persons 15–34 began to rise, especially in males, peaked during the late 1970s, and plateaued in the past decade. Its cause unexplained, the rise (lasting a generation) affected the youth of North America and many European regions (including the United Kingdom and Ireland), sparing Japan, Hong Kong, and parts of Latin America.

INTERREGIONAL DIFFERENCES

Within Canada, Newfoundland, on the Atlantic seaboard, consistently returns low regional suicide rates; and the west (chiefly Alberta and British Columbia), the highest rates (Sakinofsky, Roberts, & VanHouten, 1975). Underreporting has sometimes been suspected in Newfoundland, but scrutiny of death certificates and records is confirmatory (Aldridge & St. John, 1991). After 1969 rates in Quebec began to rise from ninth place in 1950 for males (seventh for females), to first place in 1990 for males (third for females) (Expert Working Group, 1994, pp. 30–31). Mean suicide rates for 1988–1992 are compared in Table 1 and Figure 2 (after Expert Working Group, 1994), with areas of overlap indicated by age and gender adjusted 95% confidence intervals. Male suicide is highest in the Northwest Territories, closely followed by Alberta and Quebec. Newfoundland and Ontario tie for lowest rates. A similar picture is seen for females but with more overlap in the west.

SUBPOPULATIONS

Young People

The rise of suicide in young people has been more aggressive in Canada than in the United States. To explain the youth

Isaac Sakinofsky is with the Suicide Studies Program, Clarke Institute of Psychiatry; and is Professor of Psychiatry and Preventive Medicine and Biostatistics, University of Toronto.

Antoon A. Leenaars is in private practice, Windsor, ON; and is Visiting Professor, University of Leiden, The Netherlands.

Suicide and Life-Threatening Behavior, Vol. 27(1), Spring 1997

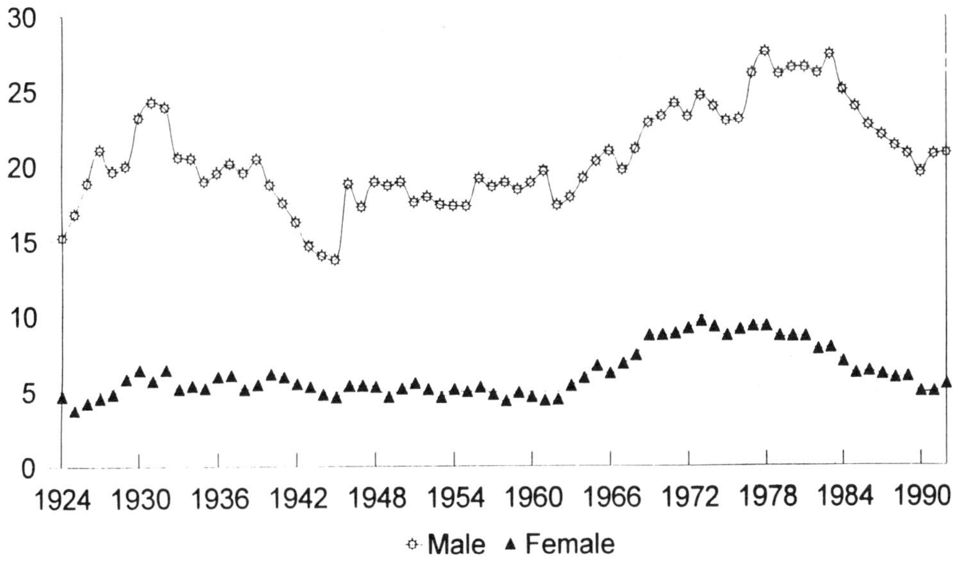

Figure 1. Crude suicide rates in Canada, 1924–1992 (aged 10 and older).

suicide rise, Klerman (1988) pointed to increased rates of depression and drug abuse, with important gender and ethnic differences. The U.S. Epidemiologic Catchment Area (ECA) study confirmed greater lifetime prevalence for major depression, schizophrenia, anxiety disorders, and alcohol abuse among younger respondents, dramatically lower in the elderly (Simon & VonKorff, 1992). Crow (1986) argued for an augmented genetic presence but this is difficult to support. Changes in society over the period are likelier explanations, with the ensuing stressors precipitating more illness and substance abuse. The end of World War II shook up the longstanding norms and values within society and weakened traditional family structures; people defected in mass from institutional religion, misused illicit psychoactive substances, radically revised the feminine role, and gave minority groups such as Blacks and gays a higher profile. All the comforting institutions of society were turned upside down. Also, the postwar baby boom, ending in the early 1960s, generated a larger birth cohort that needed to be integrated into society.

Each of these factors has been blamed. Farrow (1993) pointed out that economic recessions and unemployment "promoted the number of adolescents without a defined role in modern society . . . these are our alienated youth." These tumultuous social changes have been compared with the anomic conditions that Durkheim saw as the primary causes of suicide (Rakoff, 1983).

In Canada, rising suicide was associated with increased divorce (Leenaars, Yang, & Lester, 1993). Trovato (1992) considered the effects of divorce and religious disaffiliation more relevant than economic stress. Hasselback, Lee, Mao et al. (1991) pointed to abandonment of religion and to population proportions of (higher-risk) Native people and Francophones. A negative association with unemployment was found in this cross-sectional aggregate study, as by Sakinofsky, Roberts, and Van Houten (1975), who found 86% of the variance in male suicide explained by the percentage of persons living alone, and 89% of that for female suicide by the percentage of foreign born. Suicide correlated with other indices of social disorganization and mobility. (The failure to link it to unemployment is usual in cross-sectional but not longitudinal studies – Platt, 1984. Besides, seasonal unemployment, carried

TABLE 1
Mean Age-Adjusted Suicide Rates for Canada: Provinces and Territories, 1989–1992

Province	n/year	Mean	Confidence intervals[a] Lower	Upper
		Males		
Can	2792	20.16		
NFd	38	13.28	9.03	17.53
PEI	15	23.28	11.27	35.29
NSc	88	19.43	15.37	23.49
NBr	74	20.2	15.59	24.82
Que	902	25.63	23.95	27.3
Ont	766	14.87	13.81	15.92
Man	112	20.63	16.8	24.46
Sask	109	22.44	18.19	26.68
Alta	328	25.94	23.12	28.76
BC	336	20.07	17.92	22.22
Yuk	4	23.64	0	49.2
NWT	19	54.8	29.38	80.22
		Females		
Can	752	5.34		
NFd	6	2.14	0.44	3.85
PEI	1	1.98	0	5.46
NSc	17	3.73	1.96	5.5
NBr	13	3.34	1.49	5.2
Que	226	6.18	5.38	6.99
Ont	237	4.49	3.92	5.06
Man	27	4.88	3.01	6.73
Sask	26	5.53	3.4	7.67
Alta	97	7.81	6.24	9.38
BC	98	5.8	4.66	6.95
Yuk	1	3.42	0	12.94
NWT	3	9.17	0	19.86

[a]95% confidence intervals; direct standardization (1991 populations).

no stigma and was compensated by a "social safety net.") These ecological findings have not yet been confirmed at the individual level of investigation.

Easterlin (1980) posited that suicide rates in those of working age would be higher in a larger cohort following a smaller one because of "employment bottleneck." This theory was supported by a longitudinal study of changes in suicide rates in Canadian provinces in relation to 122 ecological variables (Sakinofsky & Roberts, 1987). Leenaars and Lester (1996) calculated positive correlations between cohort size and suicide in males aged 20–34 but not females. In the United States, Ahlburg and Schapiro (1984) found positive associations between suicide and larger cohorts of both men and women aged 15–44.

In Quebec, a region where suicide rates have increased substantially, particularly in young men, a longitudinal aggregate study showed a positive association between suicide in males 15–44 and unemployment, but only part of the period with female unemployment (Cormier & Klerman, 1985). The study cited Quebec's "quiet revolution" (greater modernism and secularism) beginning in the 1960s, which had encouraged anomie, also noted by Krull and Trovato (1994).

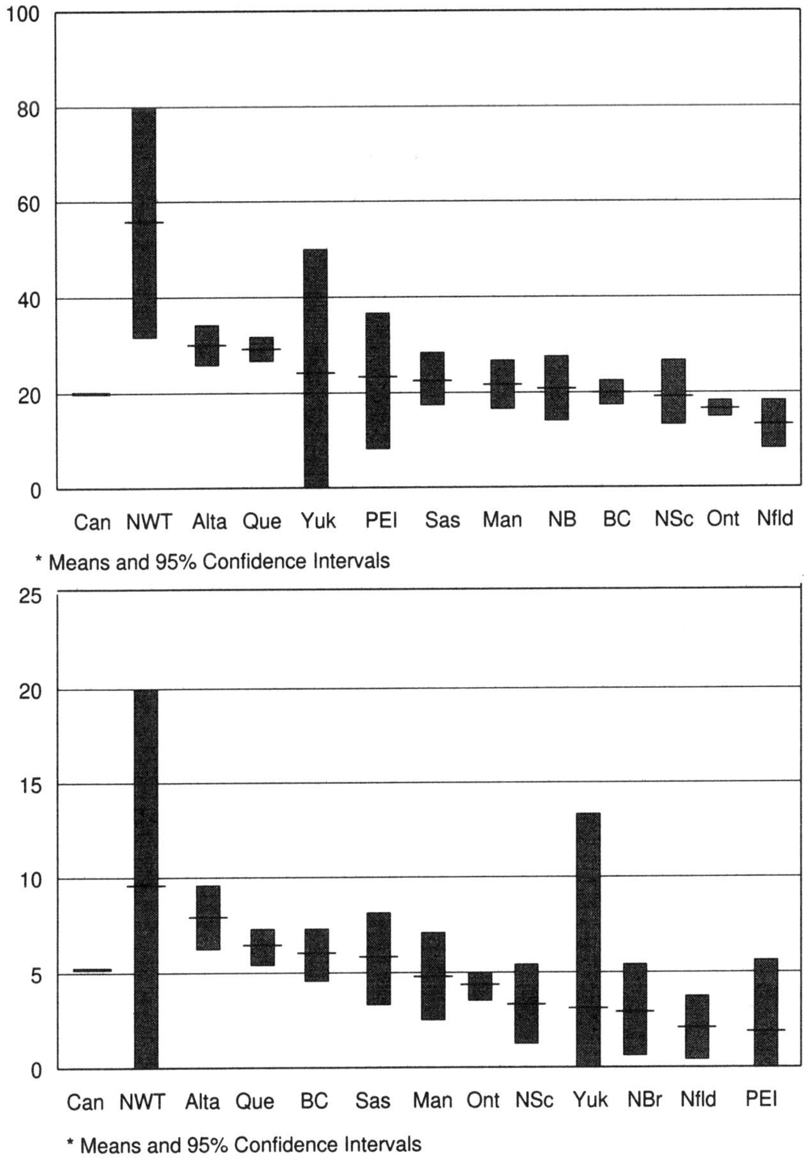

Figure 2. Rank order of suicide rates (1989–1992): Canada, Provinces, and Territories. Top: males. Bottom: females.

Aboriginal Suicide

Canada's aboriginal peoples, numbering a million, comprise 3.6% of the total population (Kirmayer, 1994); their suicide rate is 2–4 times higher than in the general population, even higher in some communities (LaRose, 1989; Sigurdson, Staley, Matas et al., 1994). Abandonment of traditional values has been blamed but it is clear that the roots of the problem are, even more, anomic. Bagley (1991) replicated an American study in 26 Native reservations in Alberta and found that in males aged 15–34 poverty and suicide were closely correlated. Gotowiec and Beiser (1994) found that Native children experience higher rates of school failure, encounter more risk of substance abuse and family violence, and are more likely to take their own lives than children in the broader culture. Gartrell, Jarvis, and Derksen (1993) studied children in the seventh to ninth grades living on Reserves and found frequent family disruption, often with a suicide already in the family. The children were depressed and their parasuicidal acts were more often fatal. Spaulding (1986) noted the lethal combination of firearms and alcohol as death factors in adolescent suicide among the Ojibway of Ontario; and Tonkin (1984), in British Columbian natives. Parasuicide in adolescent females using nonpsychotropic agents is also widespread (Ross & Davis, 1986). Hardly any of the youngsters had previous contact with mental health agencies. Suicide rates among aboriginal persons not living on Reserves were similar to the general population, and those Reserves with high suicide rates had markedly less healthy population characteristics than those with low (Cooper, Corradio, Karlberg et al., 1992).

Although data are more difficult to obtain from Inuit communities, their suicide rates are reported to be as high, and the causes similar, to those of First nations peoples (Expert Working Group, 1994). Santé Québec has sponsored several studies of suicidal behavior among aboriginal people in the north (Boyer, D., Dufour, Préville et al., 1994a; Boyer, Préville, & Legare, 1994b). 34% of Inuit aged 14–25 surveyed by Kirmayer, Malus, & Boothroyd (1996) reported a previous suicide attempt and 26% had experienced suicidal ideation within the past month. *Choosing Life*, the report of the Royal Commission on Aboriginal Peoples (1995) emphasizes the effects of demoralization caused by colonization.

METHODS USED IN SUICIDE

Death factor is a term adopted by coroners for the method of suicide. Table 2 shows how death factors have changed for male and female suicides over the decade. Suicides by firearms and drug poisonings have fallen at the expense of hanging and gassing.

Huchcroft and Tanney (1988) analyzed sex-specific suicide rates in Canada between 1971 and 1985, and commented on their divergence, male rates rising while female rates fell. Drug overdoses were declining in females and hanging, strangulation and suffocation increasing in males. In Quebec, Cheifetz, Posener, LaHaye et al. (1987) found that hanging, firearms, and jumping were the most common methods among boys aged 10–19; and drug intoxications, firearms, and jumping among girls. Between 1954 and 1980, 207 persons committed suicide and 223 unsuccessfully attempted to kill themselves under Toronto's subway trains (Johnston & Waddell, 1984). Shkrum and Johnston (1992) examined 32 deaths in Ontario from self-immolation in the period 1986–1988; half had diagnosed psychiatric illness and many had warned of their intention.

Controversy (Hung, 1993; Mundt, 1990; Sakinofsky, 1995; Whitemore, 1995) surrounded 1995 legislation in Canada for firearm registration and control (Bill C-68). Rich, Young, Fowler et al. (1990) investigated suicide methods in To-

TABLE 2
Methods Used for Suicide

	Deaths, *n* (%)	
	1980–1982	1990–1992
	Males	
Guns, explosives	3218 (41.1)	3019 (35.6)
Hanging	1920 (24.5)	2612 (30.8)
Poisoning	844 (10.8)	811 (9.6)
Gases	843 (10.8)	991 (11.7)
Jumping	321 (4.1)	372 (4.4)
Drowning	333 (4.3)	266 (3.1)
Cutting	141 (1.8)	159 (1.9)
Other	210 (2.7)	241 (2.9)
Total	7830 (100)	8471 (100)
	Females	
Guns, explosives	277 (11.3)	195 (8.8)
Hanging	463 (18.9)	492 (22.3)
Poisoning	993 (40.5)	827 (37.4)
Gases	198 (8.1)	253 (11.5)
Jumping	157 (6.4)	150 (6.8)
Drowning	208 (8.5)	156 (7.1)
Cutting	43 (1.2)	37 (1.7)
Other	115 (4.7)	100 (4.5)
Total	2454 (100)	2210 (100)

ronto and Ontario before and after the earlier (1978) Canadian gun control legislation. They concluded that substitution by jumping canceled out the beneficial effects of fewer firearm suicides, but Lester and Leenaars (1993) and Carrington and Moyer (1994a) found a significant negative trend during the postlegislation period for firearm suicide without displacement to other methods. Regional gun ownership correlated with overall suicide rates (Carrington & Moyer, 1994b). Leonard (1994) noted that guns were available in one quarter of Canadian homes.

NONFATAL SUICIDALITY

Attempted suicide stopped being reportable 30 years ago. Specialized treatment programs based in general hospitals but reaching out into the community have been in existence in Canada for a generation (Howe & Sakinofsky, 1979; Syer, 1975). The first of these was established in 1969 and modeled on the Edinburgh unit developed by Kreitman and Mathew (Kreitman, 1977; Sakinofsky, 1973). A prospective study of prevalence of treated parasuicide reported a crude rate of 730 per 100,000 per annum, several times that described elsewhere in North America (Jarvis & Boldt, 1982). The study was unusually thorough in canvassing all community agencies. Sakinofsky, Roberts, Brown et al. (1990), in hospital-treated parasuicides, obtained an annual rate of 304 per 100,000, similar to figures from Europe and the United States. Bland, Newman, and Dyck (1994) prospectively examined the records of all parasuicides who attended all Edmonton, Alberta, hospitals over one year (Bland, Dyck, Newman et al., 1995). The event incidence was 466 per 100,000 per year for persons 15 and older, with a female:male ratio of 1.6: 1. In the 15-24 age group these rates were higher than reported by most European centers (Kerkhof, Schmidtke, Bille-Brahe et al., 1994).

Community surveys are more likely than hospital-based surveys to obtain a truer estimate of nonfatal suicidality (suicidal ideation or attempts). In Calgary, Bagley and Ramsay (1985) in adults found the lifetime (one year) prevalences as follows: life not worth living, 37% (8.5%); seriously thought of or planned suicide, 13.4% (4%); parasuicide, 5.9% (1.3%); attempted suicide, 4.2% (0.8%). Dyck, Bland, Newman et al. (1988), in a larger survey in Edmonton, estimated the lifetime prevalence of suicide attempts as 3.6% (males 1.8%, and females 5.5%).

In Quebec, l'enquête Santé discovered in those 15 or more a high one year period prevalence of nonfatal suicidality of 0.8% (equivalent to a rate of 840 per 100,000). This represents a nonfatal attempt: fatal suicide ratio of 49:1. However, the one-year prevalence of ideation was only 3.9% (Emond, Guyon, Camirand et al., 1988). This compares with an Ontario survey that interviewed a sample of 9953 householders. The lifetime (one-year) prevalence of suicidal ideation was 10.7% (3.4%), and of suicide attempts 3.3% (0.4%) (Sakinofsky & Webster, 1995). The attempted suicide:competed suicide ratio was 26:1 compared with suicide data from the Chief Coroner of Ontario, lower than the Quebec estimate. The Ontario findings are similar to those of the ECA study (Moscicki, O'Carroll, Rae et al., 1988; Petronis, Samuels, Moscicki et al., 1990) and those for lifetime suicide attempt prevalence are within the international range shown in Table 3 (modified from Angst, Degonda, Ernst et al., 1992).

COMPARISONS BETWEEN CANADA AND THE UNITED STATES

Comparisons between the United States and Canada often emphasize that violence is more prevalent in the United States, (Lipset, 1990). Plainly, this is incorrect: homicides are more frequent (Leenaars & Lester, 1994) but not suicide, an internally directed form of violence. Early studies comparing suicide rates between the two countries suggested no differences as recently as the 1970s (Labovitz &

TABLE 3
Lifetime Attempts[a]

	N	%
Schwab et al. ('72)	1,645	2.7
Paykel et al. ('74)	720	1.1
Ramsey & Bagley ('85)	679	4.2
Velez & Cohen ('88)	724	3.5
Schepank ('87)	600	5.3
Dyck et al. ('88)	3,258	3.6
Moscicki et al. ('88)	18,571	2.9
Levy & Deykin ('89)	424	3.5
Breslau et al. ('91)	1,007	5.2
Wacker ('91)	470	4.7
Angst et al. ('92)	591	3.8
Bronisch et al. ('94)	481	4.1
Sakinofsky & Webster ('95)	9,943	3.3

[a]Modified from Angst et al. (1992).

Brinkerhoff, 1977). More recent studies (Leenaars & Lester, 1992a; Sakinofsky & Roberts, 1987) suggest the opposite.

Leenaars and Lester (1992b) studied the patterns of suicide in Canada and the United States during 1960–1988 using data from the National Center for Health Statistics and Statistics Canada. Until 1971 rates for both sexes were lower in Canada, but from 1977 Canadian rates (indicative of internalized violence) exceeded those in the United States.

Since 1960 rates for men in both nations have trended upwards, with a recent decrease in Canada since 1983. For women, the suicide rates in both nations appeared to be decreasing during the 1980s. Predictions that suicide in women would increase as women supposedly gained more equal social and economic equality with men (Lester, 1979) have not been realized in either country (Fig. 3).

Figure 4 presents the changing patterns of suicide by age for Canada and the United States. For both nations, rates for 3-year periods were averaged 20 years apart: 1963–1965 and 1983–1985. Both Canada and the United States experienced a tremendous increase in the suicide rates for men aged 15–34 during this period. The rise was especially notable in those aged 20–24 (i.e., young adults), whose rates shifted from the unimodal (one peak) pattern in the early 1960s to a bimodal (two-peak) pattern in the early 1980s. Peaks occur in the 20–24 group and the elderly. The results concur with recent observations by McGinnis (1987) in the United States that young adult males are a very high-risk group for suicide.

The data thus show that the suicide rates of late adolescents and young adults for both sexes in both countries have increased dramatically since 1960, especially in Canada. The rates for Canadian males aged 15–19 at times reached 50–60% higher than in the United States. Young adults, however, have an even higher rate than late adolescents, and males in this age group are most at risk. The rates for young adult males in both countries are now at the same levels as those for late adulthood. Alarmingly, the data indicate that rates in both countries have plateaued rather than subsided. For women (see Fig. 4), the patterns have remained unimodal, with a peak in middle age, for both nations and both eras.

The results show clearly that the rates and patterns of suicide in Canada and the United States are somewhat different; yet when comparison extends to other countries, their similarities are brought into focus (Cantor, Leenaars, Lester et al., 1996). Several explanations are possible for the variation in suicide patterns between the United States and Canada including variations in certification methods (O'Carroll, 1989). Researchers justifiably question the accuracy of the statistics in both countries and call for improvements (Jobes, Berman and Josselson, 1987; National Task Force on Suicide, 1987). Sainsbury and Jenkins (1982) showed that intranational comparisons are more reliable than are international comparisons of absolute rates, but the steeper trend for younger male suicide in Canada than the United States clearly validates the conclusion of more drastic increase.

Neither Canada nor the United States is a homogeneous country; each varies considerably between its counties, provinces, or states. Within both countries there are high-risk groups (e.g., aboriginal people)

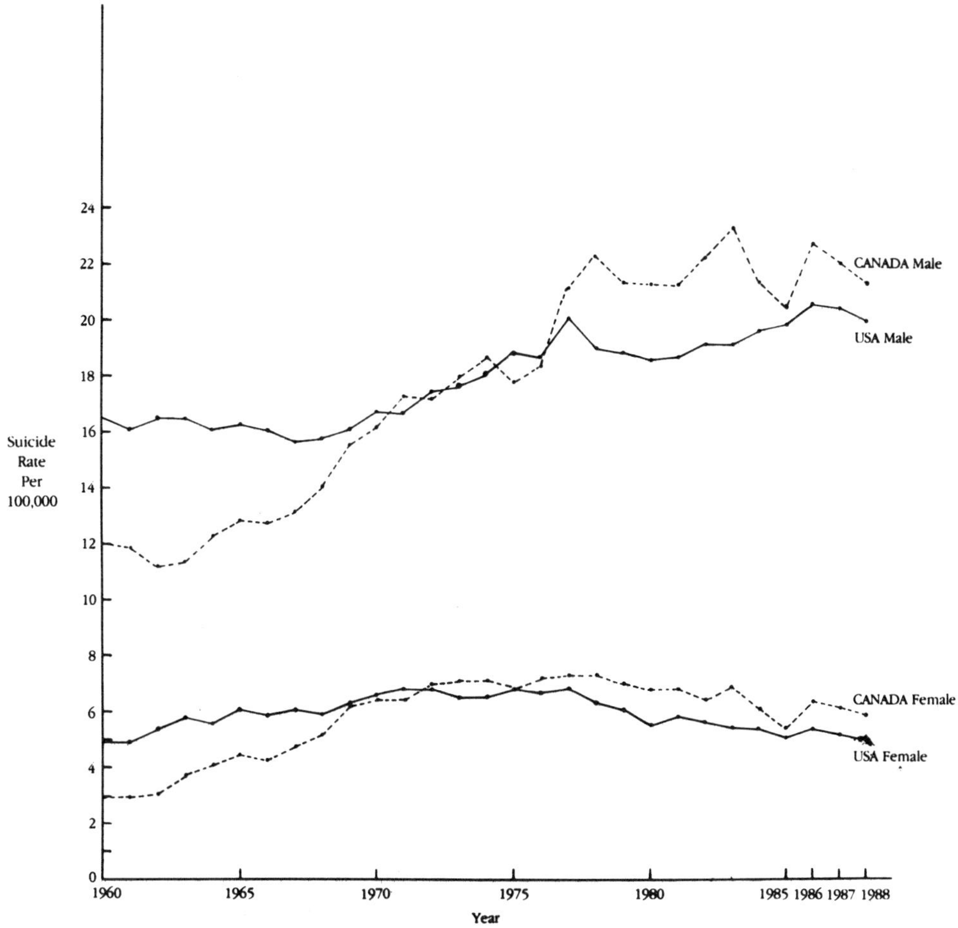

Figure 3. Suicide rates in Canada and the United States, 1960–1988.

and low-risk groups (African North Americans) for suicide. This need not vitiate the utility of comparisons between them.

Knowledge

How may we explain the probable differences between suicide in these two neighbors? Misconceptions might influence attitudes towards suicide and thus suicide rates (Shneidman & Mandelkorn, 1970). Do Canadians or Americans have greater misconceptions about suicide?

Leenaars and Lester (1992b) investigated level of knowledge about suicide of students in the United States and Canada. A knowledge questionnaire developed by Leenaars (Leenaars, Saunders, Balance et al., 1991) from Shneidman's clinically formulated facts and myths was used, consisting of 16 randomized true and false statements; for example, once a person is suicidal, he/she is suicidal forever. Overall, there was no difference in the level of correct knowledge: 83% in the Canadian and 82% in the American students. Knowledge per se (or some other measure of educational awareness) thus has little to do with varying rates.

Psychological Factors

Multidimensional viewpoints have been presented by Shneidman (1985) and Leenaars (1996). The essence of these two the-

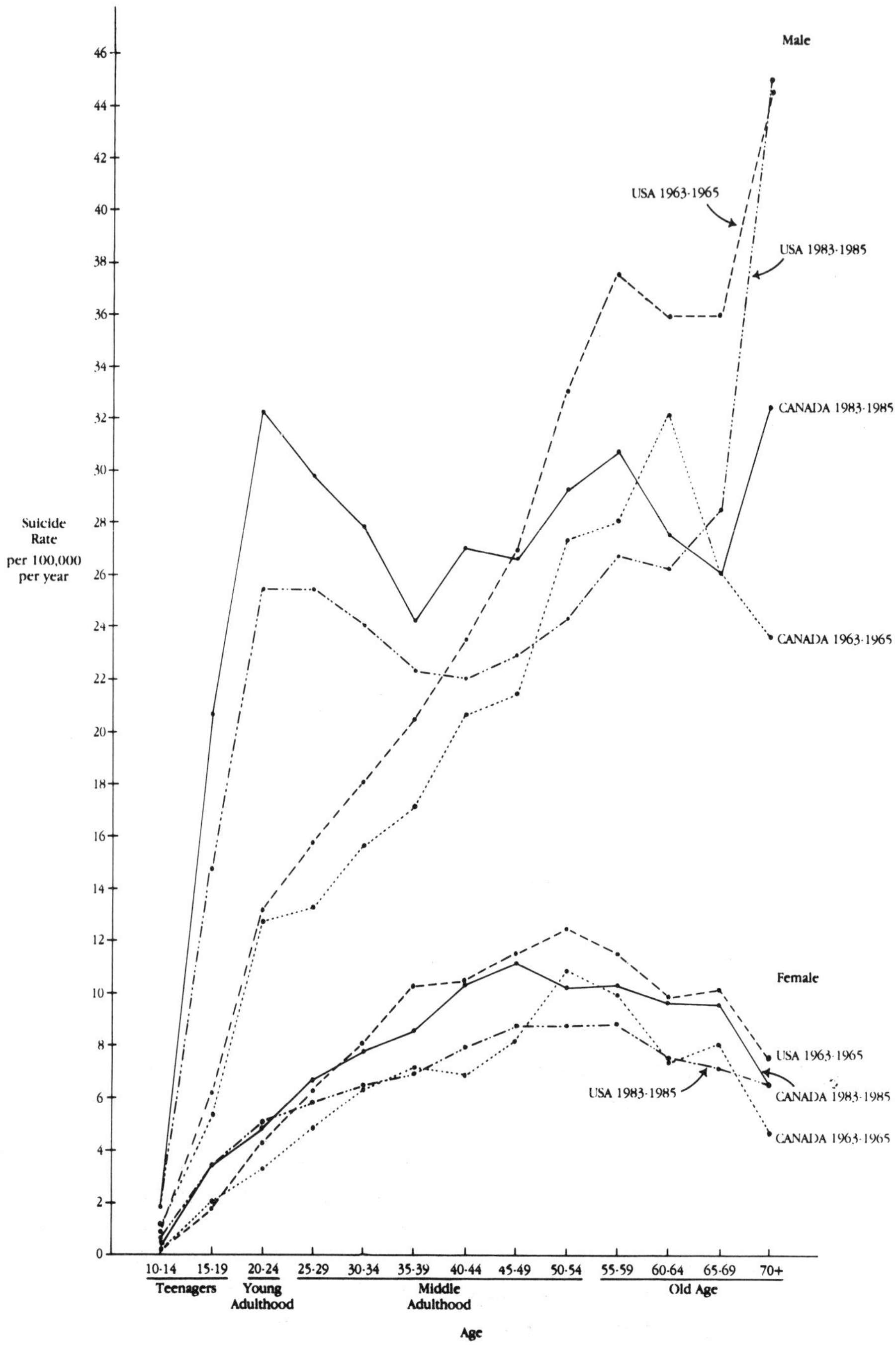

Figure 4. Suicide rates by age.

ories is that suicide is related to multidimensional psychological factors (e.g., unbearable pain, mental constriction, lost relationships). Leenaars (1992) applied this model to suicide in Canada and the United States, comparing 56 suicide notes whose writers were matched for age and sex, from both countries. No differences were noted. He concluded that this probably also eliminated differences at a psychological level, closing in on the social-cultural level.

Domestic and Economic Correlates

Durkheim (1897/1951) proposed that suicide rates were affected by two social characteristics. Suicide rates are high when the degree of social integration (the extent to which members of the society are bound together in social relationships) is very low (leading to *egoistic suicide*) or very high (leading to *altruistic suicide*). Suicide rates are also high when the degree of social regulation (the degree to which the desires and behaviors of the members of the society are controlled by societal norms and customs) is very low (leading to *anomic suicide*) or very high (leading to *fatalistic suicide*). Sociologists have noted that altruistic and fatalistic suicide are rare in modern industrialized societies, and that it is difficult to measure social regulation empirically separately from social integration. Thus, one modern version of Durkheim's theory (Johnson, 1965) states that societal suicide rates are higher when the degree of social integration/regulation is lower.

Leenaars, Yang, and Lester (1993) explored the relationship between measures of social integration/regulation and the suicide rate in both Canada and the United States for the same time period, as well as the impact of economic stress on suicide (United Nations, annuals a & b, 1950–1985). The Pearson correlations between the social and economic measures and the suicide rates of Canada and the United States are shown in Table 4, together with the results of the regression analysis. The time series regression analysis was carried out with Doan (1990) using the Cochrane–Orcutt method to correct for serial autocorrelation.

Table 4 shows that divorce rates were positively associated, and birth rates negatively associated with suicide rates, in both the simple correlational analysis and in the regression analysis for both Canada and the United States. Thus, social integration (operationally measured by low divorce rates and high birth rates) seems to be inversely associated with suicide rates in both Canada and the United States, as Durkheim predicted.

Marriage rates were positively correlated with suicide in the United States and not in Canada, but the positive U.S. association became negative on regression analysis, indicating that marriage may protect against suicide once other variables are taken into account. Unemployment was positively correlated with suicide rates for both nations but was no longer significant in the regression analysis, suggesting that unemployment adds little predictive power, and that domestic stress is a greater predictor of societal suicide rates. The protective role of family in suicide in Canada has been noted by Sakinofsky, Roberts, and VanHouten (1975). Durkheim's (1897/1951) theory appears to be useful in understanding suicide in both countries. Social integration/regulation appears related to suicide rates both in Canada and the United States. Further, Leenaars and Lester (1995) found that domestic integration (divorce, birth rates) and the economy (unemployment) better predicted youth than adult suicide rates from 1965 to 1985 in Canada. Over the same period there was less age-group variation in suicide prediction in the United States. These results call for further investigation into Canada's youth suicide problem (Leenaars & Lester, 1995).

Attitudes

Attitudes are organizing principles of values and behavior. Gordon Allport (1966) defined an attitude as "a mental and neural state of readiness, organized through experience, exerting a directive or dynamic influence upon the individual's response to all objects and situations with which it is related" (p. 20). Recent research (Diekstra, 1996) on attitudes to suicide suggests they may strongly influence the variation of suicide across the world. Domino and Leenaars (1989) and Leenaars

TABLE 4
Associations Between Measures of Domestic and Economic Stress and Suicide Rates in Canada and the United States

	Canada		United States	
	Pearson r	Regression b	Pearson r	Regression b
Divorce rate	0.97**	1.758**	0.90**	0.431**
Marriage rate	0.06	0.292	0.56**	−0.370*
Birth rate	−0.93**	−0.196**	−0.90**	−0.151**
Unemployment rate	0.73**	0.099	0.49*	−0.001

*Two-tailed $p < .01$.
**Two-tailed $p < .001$.

and Domino (1993) examined attitudes in college students and also in the more general population, discussed as follows. Using the Suicide Opinion Questionnaire (SOQ) (Domino, Moore, Westlake et al., 1982), a cross-cultural instrument (Domino & Takahashi, 1991), the results suggest significant differences between samples from Canada and the United States, both in the general population and in college students. The differences were:

- *Mental illness.* This scale assesses the attitude that suicide and mental illness are related. The general Canadian respondents and students scored significantly higher on the Mental illness scale than the U.S. groups.
- *Cry for help.* The Cry for help scale assesses the attitude that suicide represents a cry for help rather than a wish to end one's life. The Canadian general respondents also scored higher on this scale; earlier Domino and Leenaars (1989) found that both Canadian and American college students scored in a similar range.
- *Right to die.* The Right to die scale assesses the attitude that individuals do or do not have the right to terminate their own life. Again, the Canadian respondents scored higher than the U.S. respondents, a pattern congruent with that reported from college students.
- *Religion.* This scale assesses that suicide reflects the lack of religious value. Here the American respondents obtained a significantly higher mean. However, the reverse was true for students, Canadian college students scoring higher than their U.S. peers.
- *Moral evil.* This scale assesses that suicide is a morally reprehensible action. Canadian general respondents and students obtained significantly lower means than their U.S. counterparts on the Moral evil scale.
- *Normality.* Normality assesses that suicide is basically a normal action. Canadian and American general respondents equally embraced the attitude that suicide is a normal action. However, Canadian college students considered suicide normal more often than their American peers.

Clearly, their attitudinal differences do not obscure similarities that exist between attitudes towards suicide of samples of Canadians and Americans. Moreover, individual attitudes to suicide are liable to be exceedingly complex. However, the findings support the conclusion that attitudes toward suicide between Canada and the United States are not synonymous.

HISTORICAL SPECULATION ON THE CONTINENTAL DIVIDE

Max Weber (1949), a father of modern sociology, was one of the first to posit that in order to understand current events, one has to search the history. Examining the historical origins of both countries, we discover how these nations came to differ in their values and behavior. The Canadian scholar S. D. Clark (1962) noted that, "Whereas the American nation was a product of the revolutionary spirit, the Canadian nation grew mainly out of forces of a counter-revolution" (pp. 190–191). Differences between Canada and the United States could best be explained by how they settled their respective frontiers. The Canadians moved westward under the aegis of the British Government, cover of military police, and the sanction of the Roman Catholic and Anglican Churches. In contrast, America's frontier was independently settled, not as an "outpost of the empire." Canada remained loyal to Britain; the United States was born out of a revolution against her. The revolutionary attitude in the United States was distinct from a more conservative attitude in Canada. This explanation, according to Clark and others (Lipset, 1990), best accounts for the divergence in the two nations. It developed "the continental divide," the difference between Canada and the United States.

One of Canada's most celebrated novelists, Margaret Atwood (1972, 1984), suggests that the symbol for the United States is "the Frontier", "a place that is *new*, where the old can be discarded." The American revolution divided the new from the old. In Canada the symbol is "Survival," a place where one is "hanging on, staying alive." Canadians hang on to Britain (and in Quebec, to France). In her intriguing book *Survival* (1972), she writes:

> Canadians are forever taking the national pulse like doctors at a sickbed. The aim is not to see whether the patient will live well but simply whether he will live at all. Our central idea is one which generates, not the excitement and sense of adventure or danger which The Frontier holds out, not the smugness and/or sense of security, of everything in its place . . . but an almost intolerable anxiety. (p. 33)

Analyses of art, politics, religion, and maybe suicide lead to the same conclusion: There is a continental divide in values and behavior.

CONCLUSION

Epidemiological studies in Canada help us understand the extent and distribution of Canada's significant problem with suicide. Canadian subpopulations such as youth and aboriginal people are especially at risk. From an international perspective, suicide rates in Canada are unacceptably high, and suicide in youth and other at-risk groups need to be vigorously targeted. Canada's repeated efforts at gun control, one productive avenue of suicide prevention, are unfortunately unlikely to occur in the United States (Leenaars, 1995) because of cultural attitudes to freedom to bear arms (and a strong gun lobby).

Canada and the United States share close proximity, similar languages, and cultural backgrounds, and even similar suicide prevention movements. They have been open to continental comparisons in art, literature, politics, religion, etc. (Lipset, 1990). Divergence has been observed in recognition of authority, patterns of deviance, and patterns of association (Spencer, 1985). For suicide there may be more similarities between them, but despite these, differences have also been observed in families and attitudes to suicide, including issues of the right to die. Each nation is unique and the two gain when they pool their understanding of suicide and its prevention.

Research informs such understanding, but Maris (1993) noted that very little funding for research into suicide is available in America. Canada's problem is even worse (Leenaars, 1995), its per capita support for research among the lowest in major countries reporting to the Organization for Economic Cooperation and Development (Lipset, 1990). Support has declined progressively since the 1970s. Government funding agencies have few resources for suicide research, and there is no Canadian equivalent of the American

Suicide Foundation (or for the granting bodies that exist for many mental and physical disorders). It is grimly unfortunate that both Canada and the United States, with their serious suicide problems, lack a tradition of support for research into suicide.

REFERENCES

Ahlburg, D., & Schapiro, M. (1984). Socioeconomic ramifications of changing cohort size: An analysis of U.S. postwar suicide rates by age and sex. *Demography, 21*, 97–108.

Aldridge, D., & St. John, K. (1991). Adolescent and pre-adolescent suicide in Newfoundland and Labrador. *Canadian Journal of Psychiatry, 36*, 432–436.

Allport, G. (1966). Attitudes in the history of social psychology. In M. Jahoda & N. Warren (Eds.), *Attitudes.* New York: Penguin. (original published in 1954).

Angst, J., Degonda, M., & Ernst, C. (1992). The Zurich study: XV. Suicide attempts in a cohort from age 20 to 30. *European Archives of Psychiatry & Clinical Neuroscience, 242*, 135–141.

Atwood, M. (1972). *Survival.* Toronto: Anasi.

Atwood, M. (1984). *Second words: Selected critical prose.* Boston: Beacon Press.

Bagley, C. (1991). Poverty and suicide among Native Canadians: A replication. *Psychological Reports, 69*, 149–150.

Bagley, C., & Ramsay, R. (1985). Psychosocial correlates of suicidal behaviours in an urban population. *Crisis, 6*, 63–77.

Bland, R., Newman, S., & Dyck, R. (1994). The epidemiology of parasuicide in Edmonton. *Canadian Journal of Psychiatry, 39*, 391–396.

Bland, R., Dyck, R., Newman, S., & Om, H. (1995, September). *Parasuicide in Edmonton.* Presented at the Canadian Academy of Psychiatric Epidemiology Meeting, Victoria, BC.

Boyer, R., Dufour, R., Préville, M., & Bujold-Brown, L. (1994a). State of mental health. In Santé Québec (Ed.), *A health profile of the Inuit. Report of the Santé Québec health survey among the Inuit of Nunavik, 1992* (pp. 117–144) Montréal: Ministère de la Santé et Service sociaux, Gouvernement du Québec.

Boyer, R., Préville, M., & Légaré, G. (1994b). Mental Health. In Santé Québec (Ed.), *A health profile of the Cree. Report of the Santé Québec health survey of the James Bay Cree, 1991* (pp. 161–173). Montréal: Ministère de la Santé et Service sociaux, Gouvernement du Québec.

Brown, J. (1975). Reporting of suicide: Canadian statistics. *Suicide, 5*, 21–28.

Cantor, C., Leenaars, A., Lester, D., Slatter, P., Wolanowski, T., & O'Toole, B. (1996). Suicide trends in eight predominately English-speaking countries (1960–1989). *Social Psychiatry and Psychiatric Epidemiology, 31*, 364–373.

Carrington, P., & Moyer, S. (1994a). Gun control and suicide in Ontario. *American Journal of Psychiatry, 151*, 606–608.

Carrington, P., & Moyer, S. (1994b). Gun availability and suicide in Canada: Testing the displacement hypothesis. *Studies on Crime & Crime Prevention, 3*, 168–178.

Cheifetz, P., Posener, J., LaHaye, A., Zajdman, M., et al. (1987). An epidemiological study of adolescent suicide. *Canadian Journal of Psychiatry, 32*, 656–659.

Clark, S. (1962). *The developing Canadian community.* Toronto: University of Toronto Press.

Cooper, M., Corradio, R., Karlberg, A., & Adams, L. (1992). Aboriginal suicide in British Columbia: An overview. *Canada's Mental Health, 40*, 19–23.

Cormier, H., & Klerman, G. (1985). Unemployment and male labour force participation as determinants of changing suicide rates of males and females in Quebec. *Social Psychiatry, 20*, 109–114.

Crow, T. J. (1986). Secular changes in affective disorder and variations in the psychosis gene. *Archives of General Psychiatry, 43*, 1013–1014.

Diekstra, R. (1996). *International perspectives.* Keynote paper, American Association of Suicidology Meeting, St. Louis.

Doan, T. (1990). *Regression analysis of time series.* Evanston, IL: Var Econometrics.

Domino, G., & Leenaars, A. (1989). Attitudes towards suicide: A comparison of Canadian and United States college students. *Suicide and Life-Threatening Behavior, 19*, 160–172.

Domino, G., MacGregor, J., & Hannah, M. (1988–89). Collegiate attitudes toward suicide: New Zealand and United States. *Omega, 19*, 351–364.

Domino, G., Moore, D., Westlake, L., & Gibson, L. (1982). Attitudes towards suicide: A factor analytic approach. *Journal of Clinical Psychology, 38*, 257–262.

Domino, G., & Takahashi, Y. (1991). Attitudes towards suicide in Japanese and American medical students. *Suicide & Life-Threatening Behavior, 21*, 345–359.

Durkheim, E. (1951). *Suicide* (J. Spaulding & G. Simpson, Trans.). Glencoe IL: The Free Press. (Original published in 1897)

Dyck, R., Bland, R., Newman, S., & Orn, H. (1988). Suicide attempts and psychiatric disorder in Edmonton. *Acta Psychiatrica Scandinavica, 77* (Suppl. 338), 64–71.

Easterlin, R. (1980). *Birth and fortune: The impact of numbers on personal welfare.* New York: Basic Books.

Emond, A., Guyon, L., Camirand, F., Chenard, L., Pineault, R., & Robitaille, Y. (1988). *Et La Sante, ca va? Rapport de l'enquête Santé Québec.* Montréal: Le Publications du Québec.

Expert Working Group. (1994). *Suicide in Canada: Update of the Report of the Task Force on Suicide in Canada.* Ottawa: Minister of National Health and Welfare.

Farrow, J. (1993). Youth alienation as an emerging pediatric health care issue: update. *American Journal of Diseases of Children, 147*, 509.

Gartrell, J., Jarvis, G., & Derksen, L. (1993). Suicidality among adolescent Alberta Indians. *Suicide and Life-Threatening Behavior, 23*, 366–373.

Gotowiec, A., & Beiser, M. (1994). Aboriginal children's mental health: Unique challenges. *Canada's Mental Health, 41*, 7–11.

Hasselback, P., Lee, K., Mao, Y., Nichol, R., & Wigle, D. (1991). The relationship of suicide rates to sociodemographic factors in Canadian census divisions. *Canadian Journal of Psychiatry, 36*, 655-659.

Health & Welfare Canada. (1992). *Aboriginal health in Canada.* Ottawa: Ministry of Supply & Services.

Howe, A., & Sakinofsky, I. (1979). A short-stay intensive care multidisciplinary unit for parasuicide. *10th International Congress for Suicide Prevention & Crisis Intervention, 2*, 34-38.

Huchcroft, S., & Tanney, B. (1988). Sex-specific suicide trends in Canada, 1971-1985. *International Journal of Epidemiology, 17*, 839-843.

Hung, C. (1993). "Gun control and rates of firearms violence in Canada and the United States": Comment. *Canadian Journal of Criminology, 35*, 37-41.

Jarvis, G., & Boldt, M. (1982). Death styles among Canada's Indians. *Social Science and Medicine, 16*, 1345-1352.

Jobes, P., Berman, A., & Josselson, A. (1987). Improving the validity and reliability of medical-legal certification of suicide. *Suicide & Life-Threatening Behavior, 17*, 310-325.

Johnson, D. (1965). Durkheim's one cause of suicide. *American Sociological Review, 30*, 875-886.

Johnson, D., & Waddell, J. (1984). Death and injury patterns, Toronto Subway System 1954-1980. *Journal of Trauma, 24*, 619-622.

Kehoe, J., & Abbott, A. (1975). Suicide and attempted suicide in the Yukon Territory. *Canadian Psychiatric Association Journal, 20*, 15-23.

Kerkhof, A., Schmidtke, A., Bille-Brahe, U., De Leo, D., & Lönnqvist, J. (1994). *Attempted suicide in Europe: Findings from the multicentre study of parasuicide by the WHO regional office for Europe.* Leiden: Leiden University, DSWO Press & World Health Organization.

Kirmayer, L. (1994). Suicide among Canadian Aboriginal peoples. *Transcultural Psychiatric Research Review, 31*, 3-58.

Kirmayer, L. J., Malus, M., & Boothroyd, L. J. (1996). Suicide attempts among Inuit youth: A community survey of prevalence and risk factors. *Acta Psychiatrica Scandinavica, 94*, 8-17.

Klerman, G. (1988). The current age of youthful melancholia. *British Journal of Psychiatry, 152*, 4-14.

Kreitman, N. (1977). *Parasuicide.* London: John Wiley.

Krull, C., & Trovato, F. (1994). The Quiet Revolution and the sex differential in Quebec's suicide rates: 1931-1986. *Social Forces, 72*, 1121-1147.

Labovitz, S., & Brinkerhoff, M. (1977). Structural changes and suicide in Canada. *International Journal of Comparative Sociology, 18*, 254-267.

LaRose, F. (1989). L'environnement des reserves Indiennes est-il pathogene? Reflexions sur le suicide et l'identification des facteurs de risque en milieu Amerindien Quebecois. *Revue Quebecoise de Psychologie, 10*, 31-44.

Leenaars, A. (1988). *Suicide notes.* New York: Human Sciences Press.

Leenaars, A. (1989a). Are young adults' suicides psychologically different from those of other adults? *Suicide & Life-Threatening Behavior, 19*, 249-263.

Leenaars, A. (1989b). *Rates and patterns of suicide for Canada and the United States: Their implications for sociopolitical action.* Presidential address presented at the first regional Canadian Association for Suicide Prevention Conference, Toronto.

Leenaars, A. (1992). Suicide notes from Canada and the United States. *Perceptual and Motor Skills, 74*, 278.

Leenaars, A. (1995). Suicide and the continental divide. *Archives of Suicide Research, 1*, 39-58.

Leenaars, A. (1996, in press). Suicide: A multidimensional malaise. *Suicide & Life-Threatening Behavior.*

Leenaars, A., & Lester, D. (1990). Suicide in adolescents: A comparison of Canada and the United States. *Psychological Reports, 67*, 867-873.

Leenaars, A., & Lester, D. (1992a). Comparison of rates and patterns of suicide in Canada and the United States, 1960-1988. *Death Studies, 16*, 417-430.

Leenaars, A., & Lester, D. (1992b). Facts & myths of suicide in Canada and the United States. *Journal of Social Psychology; 132*, 787-789.

Leenaars, A., & Lester, D. (1994). Suicide and homicide rates in Canada and the United States. *Suicide & Life-Threatening Behavior, 24*, 184-191.

Leenaars, A., & Lester, D. (1995). The changing suicide pattern in Canadian adolescents and youth compared to their American counterparts. *Adolescence, 30*, 539-547.

Leenaars, A., & Lester, D. (1996). Testing the cohort size hypothesis of suicide and homicide rates in Canada and the United States. *Archives of Suicide Research, 2*, 43-54.

Leenaars, A., Saunders, M., Balance, W., Wenckstern, S., & Galgan, R. (1991). Knowledge about facts and myths of suicide in the elderly. *Gerontology & Geriatrics Education, 12*, 61-68.

Leenaars, A., Yang, B., & Lester, D. (1993). The effect of domestic and economic stress on suicide rates in Canada and the United States. *Journal of Clinical Psychology, 49*, 918-921.

Leenaars, A. A., & Domino, G. (1993). Comparison of community attitudes towards suicide in Windsor and Los Angeles. *Suicide and Life-Threatening Behavior, 25*, 253-266.

Leonard, K. (1994). Firearm deaths in Canadian adolescents and young adults. *Canadian Journal of Public Health, 85*, 128-131.

Lester, D. (1972). Migration and suicide. *Medical Journal of Australia, 1*, 941-942.

Lester, D. (1979). Sex differences in suicidal behavior. In E. Gomberg & V. Franks (Eds.), *Gender and disordered behavior.* New York: Brunner/Mazel.

Lester, D., & Leenaars, A. (1993). Suicide rates in Canada before and after tightening firearm control laws. *Psychological Reports, 72*, 787-790.

Liberakis, E., & Hoenig, J. (1978). Recording of suicide in Newfoundland. *Psychiatric Journal of the University of Ottawa, 3*, 254-259.

Lipset, S. (1990). *Continental divide.* New York: Routledge.

Maris, R. (1993). The evolution of suicidology as a professional discipline. In A. Leenaars, (Ed.), *Suicidology: Essays in honor of Edwin S. Shneidman* (pp. 3-21). Northvale, NJ: Jason Aronson.

McGinnis, J. (1987). Suicide in America – moving up the public health agenda. *Suicide and Life-Threatening Behavior, 17*, 18-32.

Moscicki, E., O'Carroll, P., Rae, D., Locke, B., Roy, A., & Regier, D. (1988). Suicide attempts in the Epidemiologic Catchment Area study. *Yale Journal of Biology & Medicine, 61*, 259-268.

Mundt, R. J. (1990). Gun control and rates of firearm violence in Canada and the United States. *Canadian Journal of Criminology, 32*, 137-154.

National Center for Health Statistics. (Annual). *Vital statistics of the United States.* Washington, DC: United States Government Printing Office.

National Task Force on Suicide in Canada. (1987). *Suicide in Canada.* Ottawa: Minister of National Health and Welfare.

O'Carroll, P. (1989). A consideration of the validity and reliability of suicide mortality data. *Suicide & Life-Threatening Behavior, 18*, 1-16.

Petronis, K., Samuels, J., Moscicki, E., & Anthony, J. (1990). An epidemiological investigation of potential risk factors for suicide attempts. *Social Psychiatry & Psychiatric Epidemiology, 25*, 193-199.

Platt, S. (1984). Unemployment and suicidal behaviour: A review of the literature. *Social Science & Medicine, 19*, 93-115.

Rakoff, V. (1983). Anomic suicide: the persistence of a problem. The spectrum of antidepressant effect. *In proceedings of the VII World Congress of Psychiatry.* Vienna: World Congress of Psychiatry.

Rich, C., Young, J., Fowler, R., Wagner, J., & Black, N. (1990). Guns and suicide: possible effects of some specific legislation. *American Journal of Psychiatry, 147*, 342-346.

Ross, C., & Davis, B. (1986). Suicide and parasuicide in a northern Canadian native community. *Canadian Journal of Psychiatry, 31*, 331-334.

Royal Commission on Aboriginal Peoples. (1995). *Choosing Life. Special report on suicide among Aboriginal peoples.* Ottawa: Minister of Supply & Services Canada.

Sainsbury, P., & Jenkins, J. (1982). The accuracy of officially reported suicide statistics for the purposes of epidemiological research. *Journal of Epidemiology and Community Health, 36*, 43-48.

Sakinofsky, I. (1973). Experience of comprehensive care of attempted suicide within a general hospital. In A. Russel (Ed.), *Proceedings of the Suicide Symposium, Oxford Mental Health Centre*, Woodstock, ON.

Sakinofsky, I. (1995, July 1). The risk that available guns pose. Letter to the *Globe & Mail*, p. D7.

Sakinofsky, I., & Roberts, R. (1987). The ecology of suicide in the provinces of Canada: 1969-71 to 1979-81. In B. Cooper (Ed.), *The epidemiology of psychiatric disorders* (pp. 27-42). Baltimore: Johns Hopkins.

Sakinofsky, I., Roberts, R., Brown, Y., Cooper, C., James, P. (1990). Problem resolution and repetition of parasuicide: A prospective study. *British Journal of Psychiatry, 156*, 395-399.

Sakinofsky, I., Roberts, R., & Van Houten, A. (1975). *The end of the journey: A study of suicide across Canada.* Presented at the 8th International Congress on Suicide Prevention & Crisis Intervention, Jerusalem.

Sakinofsky, I., & Webster, G. (1995, June). *Major risk factors for non-fatal suicidality in the community.* Presented at the 18 Congress of the International Association for Suicide Prevention and Crisis Intervention (IASP), Venice.

Shkrum, M., & Johnston, K. (1992). Fire and suicide: A three year study of self immolation deaths. *Journal of Forensic Sciences, 37*, 208-221.

Shneidman, E. (1985). *Definition of suicide.* New York: Wiley.

Shneidman, E., & Mandelkorn, P. (1970). How to prevent suicide. In E. Shneidman, N. Farberow, & R. Litman (Eds.), *The psychology of suicide* (pp. 125-143). New York: Science House.

Sigurdson, E., Staley, D., Matas, M., Hildahl, K., & Squair, K. (1994). A five year review of youth suicide in Manitoba. *Canadian Journal of Psychiatry, 39*, 397-403.

Simon, G., & VonKorff, M. (1992). Reevaluation of secular trends in depression rates. *American Journal of Epidemiology, 135*, 1411-1422.

Spaulding, J. (1986). Recent suicide rates among ten Ojibway Indian bands in Northwestern Ontario. *Omega: Journal of Death and Dying, 16*, 347-354.

Spencer, M. (1985). *Foundations of modern sociology.* Scarborough, ON: Prentice Hall, Canada.

Statistics Canada. (annual). *Suicide statistics of Canada.* Ottawa: Author.

Syer, D. (1975). Emergency ward treatment of suicidal patients. *Ontario Psychologist, 7*, 33-37.

Tonkin, R. (1984). Suicide methods in British Columbian adolescents. *Journal of Adolescent Health Care, 5*, 172-177.

Trovato, F. (1987). A longitudinal analysis of divorce and suicide in Canada. *Journal of Marriage and the Family, 49*, 193-203.

Trovato, F. (1992). A Durkheimian analysis of youth suicide: Canada, 1971 and 1981. *Suicide and Life-Threatening Behavior, 22*, 413-427.

United Nations. (annual a & b, 1950-1985). *Demographic yearbook and Statistical yearbook.* Geneva: United Nations.

Weber, M. (1949). *The methodology of social sciences.* Glencoe, IL Free Press. (Original published in various years, early 20th century)

Whitemore, L. (1995, June 22). Gun Control. Letter to the *Globe & Mail.*

13
Perspective: Suicide in Europe

Armin Schmidtke, PhD

In many European countries, suicidal behavior constitutes a major public and mental health problem. In most countries, the number of suicides is significantly higher than the number of deaths due to traffic accidents. According to official figures, the suicide rates among European countries differ widely; for example, Hungary has the highest rates. Suicide attempt rates, based on data from the WHO/Euro Multicentre project on Parasuicide, equally show variation; for example, the highest average rate of suicide attempts is for Helsinki, Finland. This paper outlines the epidemiological findings and then presents some hypotheses (e.g., age, ethnic difference) to explain the differences.

In many European countries, suicidal behavior constitutes a major public and mental health problem and a considerable drain on resources in both primary and secondary health care settings (Schmidtke et al., 1996). In most counties, the number of suicides is significantly higher than the number of deaths due to traffic accidents (Diekstra, 1996). In some age groups, especially the younger age groups, suicide ranks after accidents as one of the leading causes of death (Schmidtke, 1995). Among the elderly, countries with an increase in old-age suicide outnumber those with a decrease 2:1 (Gulbinat, 1996). Suicide attempts are responsible for a high percentage of admissions in emergency units (Schmidtke et al., 1988). Therefore, in implementing the WHO program "Health for All by the Year 2000," the European region of WHO also identified prevention of suicidal behavior as a main target. In Target 12, it is stated that: "By the year 2000, there should be a sustained and continuing reduction of the current rising trends in suicide and attempted suicide" (WHO, 1992). In fulfilling these aims, efforts were made to implement prevention strategies in many European countries. Also, the WHO/EURO Multicentre Project on Parasuicide has a significant role for the implementation of Target 12 in the European region (Schmidtke, 1989; WHO, 1992). In this context, some efforts have also been made to explain the differences of suicidal behavior among the various European countries and to understand the different meanings of this behavior in the different European cultures.

SUICIDE RATES IN EUROPE

According to the latest official figures released by WHO and the individual national bureaus of statistics, the suicide rates among European countries differ widely (Wedel, 1992; WHO, 1995; see Fig. 1). However, also within a country, some regions or states – like in the former Yugoslavia (Milcinski & Mrevlje, 1990), Hungary, or Germany – often have significantly varying suicide rates (Schmidtke, 1995).

Since the beginning of official registration, Hungary has been the country with the highest suicide rates in Europe (if not in the world). The average rate for the period 1989–1993 is 58.8/100,000. Nordic and Eastern (Värnik & Wassermann, 1994) European countries also have somewhat higher suicide rates, whereas the southern parts of Europe have comparatively low suicide rates (see Fig. 2).

Armin Schmidtke is with the University of Würzburg. Address correspondence to the author at Psychiatrische Klinik, Klin Psychologie, Fuchsleit Str. 15, 97080 Würzburg, Germany.

Suicide and Life-Threatening Behavior, Vol. 27(1), Spring 1997

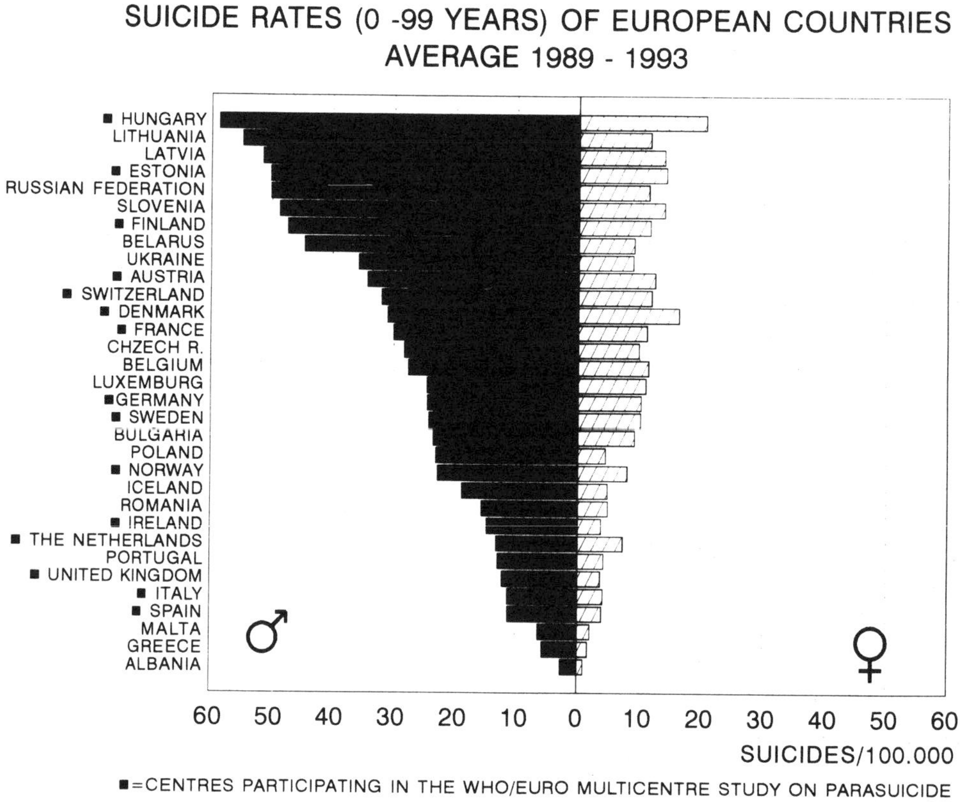

Figure 1. Suicide rates (0–99 years) of the various European countries; average 1989–1993. Source: annual figures from the WHO data bank and national bureaus of statistics. Computations of means: Department of Clinical Psychology, Psychiatric Clinic, University of Würzburg.

The average European male suicide rate is 27.9 (s = 15.6); however, there is more than 22-fold difference between the highest (Hungary) and the lowest suicide rates (Albania) for males. The average female rate is 8.9/100,000 (s = 4.6) with a 20-fold difference between the highest rate (again Hungary, with 20.7) and the lowest rate (Albania, with 1.0). In all countries, the male suicide rate is higher than the female suicide rate: the average ratio is 3.2, with the lowest male:female ratio of 1.8 in the Netherlands and the highest of 5.1 in Poland (the next highest is found for Belarus, with 4.9). Most Nordic and Eastern countries have higher male/female ratios than the western and southern countries.

The suicide methods used also differ widely. There are statistically significant preferences for methods of suicide in comparison to non-European countries also (Snyder, 1994). For example, in Germany "hanging" is the most predominant suicide method, whereas in some Nordic countries (e.g., Norway), the method "gun" is used in almost a third of all suicide methods. With regard to the drugs and poisons used, there are also great differences with regard to their toxicity. For example, the rate of using herbicides and pesticides is much higher in Hungary than in the rest of Europe.

With regard to the age distribution of suicide, one can find a "Hungarian pattern" of the suicide rates in most countries (Wedel, 1992), for example, the suicide rates increase with age (e.g., Fuse, 1980, in Lester 1982). Most correlation coefficients between suicide rates and age are positive and significant for both females and males;

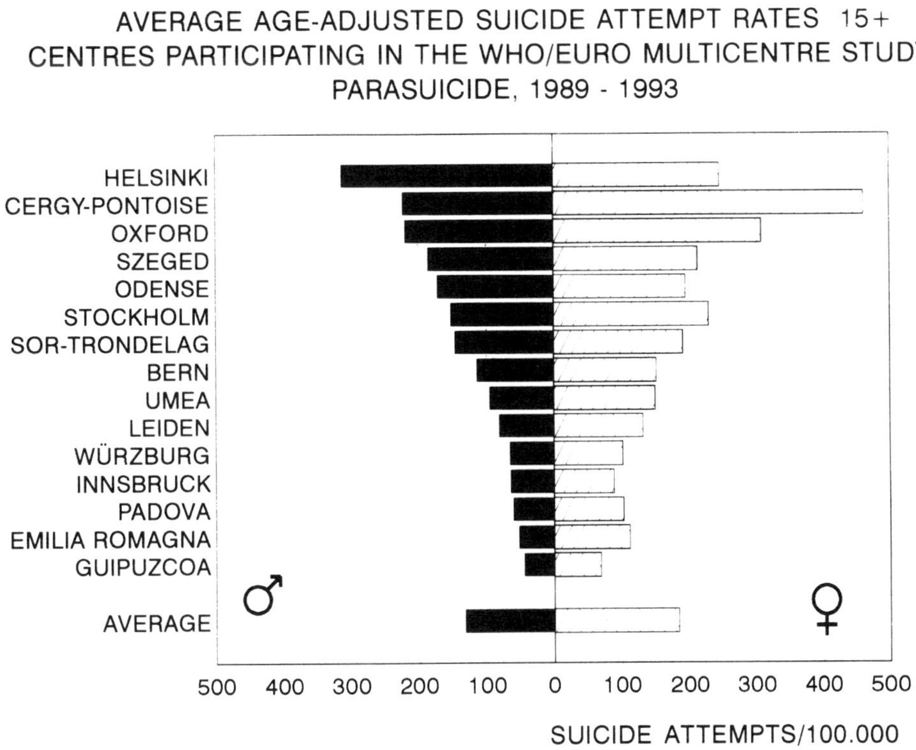

Figure 2. Suicide attempt rates in various European catchment areas. Source: WHO/EURO Multicentre Study on Parasuicide.

however, the covariation in males in most countries is more pronounced.

SUICIDE ATTEMPT RATES

Official suicide attempt rates do not exist for most European countries. Therefore, in the WHO/EURO Multicentre Project on Parasuicide, one aim is also to develop indicators for this target. Since 1989, 16 centers in 13 European countries have been trying to assess "real" suicide attempt rates and trends as well as the epidemiology of suicide attempts. In order to avoid as far as possible errors made in previous studies, a common definition of suicidal behavior is used. In this proposed International Classification of Diseases (ICD-10) definition, "parasuicide" was defined as "An act with nonfatal outcome, in which an individual deliberately initiates a non-habitual behaviour that, without intervention from others, will cause self-harm, or deliberately ingests a substance in excess of the prescribed or generally recognized therapeutic dosage, and which is aimed at realizing changes which the subject desired via the actual or expected physical consequences." To ensure that data collection was identical in all centers, a common instrument was used by all participants (Platt et al., 1992; Schmidtke et al., 1993).

The latest results show the highest average male age-standardized person rate of suicide attempts for Helsinki (Finland: 314/100,000), and the lowest (45/100,000) for Guipuzcoa (Spain). This represents a sevenfold difference. The highest average female age-standardized rate was found for Cergy-Pontoise (France: 462/100,000), and the lowest (69/100,000) again for Guipuzcoa. With only one exception (Helsinki), the person-based suicide attempt rates were higher among women than men. In the majority of centers, the highest person-based rates were found in the younger age groups. The rates among people aged 55 years or more were generally the lowest. For the majority of the centers, the rates for persons aged 15+ years decreased between 1989 and 1992 (Schmidtke et al., 1996).

The methods used were primarily "soft," such as poisoning or cutting. More than 50% of the suicide attempters committed more than one attempt, and nearly 20% of the second attempts were made within 12 months after the first attempt. Compared with the general population, suicide attempters more often belong to the social categories that indicate social destabilization and poverty.

However, if the suicide attempt rates in the centers were compared with their suicide rates 15+, the rank orders covary significantly only for males. The rank correlation coefficient is .58 ($p < .03$). The mean ratio suicide:suicide attempt for males is 1:5.3, the range being 1:2.1 (Innsbruck)–1:19.8 (Oxford) (Schmidtke et al., 1995).

For females, the rank orders for suicide attempt rates and suicide rates do not covary significantly, neither for the center nor for the country data. The rank correlation coefficient is .36 (NS). The mean ratio suicide:suicide attempt for females is 1: 21.2, the range being 1:7.8 (Szeged)–1:86 (Oxford) (Schmidtke et al., 1995).

Even though not all centers provided data for all years, where comparisons were possible, the rank order of the different centers did not change drastically over the period covered. Helsinki, Oxford, Cergy-Pontoise, Szeged, and Odense were consistently the centers with the highest rates for males. Emilia-Romagna, Guipuzcoa, Padova, and Würzburg were the centers with the lowest rates. The center with the highest female rates was always Cergy-Pontoise, the second highest was always Oxford, and the third highest rates were most often found for Helsinki. The center with the lowest rates was always Guipuzcoa. Padova, Würzburg, and Innsbruck most often had the second to fourth lowest ranks.

HYPOTHESES TO EXPLAIN THE DIFFERENCES

Reliability and Validity of Death Certification and Reporting

As a first explanation for these differences among European countries, as in other parts of the world, the question of the reliability and validity of death certification and reporting has been raised (Sainsbury, 1983; Schmidtke & Weinacker, 1991; WHO, 1982). The European countries differ widely with regard to their death certification procedures, ranging from a coroner system (United Kingdom) to the possibility that any general practitioner can sign the death certificate (Germany). Also, the rate of autopsies varies greatly with, for example, high rates in Austria and very low rates in Germany. Therefore, some studies have shown that, especially among the older age groups, there is a covariation between the number of "undetermined" deaths and the suicide figures (DeLeo, Carollo, Dello Buono, Conforti, & Mastinu, 1995; Schmidtke & Weinacker, 1991). There is no doubt that the quality and reliability of official mortality reporting varies tremendously among the various European countries. For example, in a study in an Irish county it was found that of suicides, undetermined deaths, and accidents, in all, 35% were, in the author's opinion, miscoded or unregistered. Official registration was lacking for 7.3%, the greatest miscoding was found for deaths due to drowning (Connolly & Cullen, 1995). Therefore, a direct comparison and interpretation of the differences of suicide rates among the European countries has to be made carefully. However, the analysis of trends over time or the ratios of suicide rates (e.g., such as male/female rates or old/young rates) may be less sensitive to different reporting patterns (Gulbinat, 1996).

Age Structure

A second often quoted methodological-based hypothesis is that the differences in suicide and suicide attempt rates are only caused by the different age pyramids of the different countries. However, various studies show for suicide (Diekstra, 1996) as well as for suicide attempts (Schmidtke et al., 1996) that there are no significant main differences between the crude and the age-adjusted rates.

Ethnic Differences

Because several studies show that differences in the rank order of suicide rates in the native countries covary with differences of the same cultural groups in other countries (Lester, 1972; Sainsbury & Barraclough, 1968; Schmidtke et al., 1994), the difference in ascertainment procedures do not explain all differences in the suicide rates between the various European countries (e.g., Diekstra, 1996). Another proof for this assumption is that Hungary, Saxonia, and Thuringia, regardless of their government, have consistently had higher suicide rates than the rest of Europe and Germany.

Historically some authors have published the hypothesis that the suicide rates in areas with more "Germanic" population is higher than in regions with more Romanic or Slavic populations (Morselli, 1881). These hypotheses were also used to explain, for example, the constant differences of suicide rates within Germany. Still in 1960, Winkler explained this with the "known tendency of the Saxonian–Thuringian population toward suicide"; and he added, "since other factors can be excluded this must be due to their 'character'" (Winkler, 1960, p. 144).

Today the hypotheses with regard to these ethnic differences are numerous, ranging from biological hypotheses to nutrition and attitude factors. However, no sufficient explanation is available to convincingly account for these differences with biological factors.

Methodologically profound studies also show that these differences in suicide rates between the countries are not equally distributed for all age groups. Most differences are (even for the states or areas within one country) only significant for the older age groups (Moksony, 1995; Schmidtke, 1995).

Sociodemographic Explanations

Despite the fact that many studies show a covariation of certain primarily negative sociodemographic or socioeconomic conditions and the occurrence of at least attempted suicide (Platt & Kreitman, 1985; Platt, 1986; Rygnestad & Hauge, 1991; Schmidtke et al., 1996), simple sociodemographic explanations (e.g., different unemployment rates, different participation of women in the labor force, and social security systems) also do not explain the variations in European suicide and suicide attempt rates. Whereas the unemployment rate was increasing in the United Kingdom in the 1970s, the suicide rates decreased. Although the unemployment rate in the eastern parts of Germany has increased and is significantly higher than before (officially, the German Democratic Republic did not have unemployed citizens), the suicide rates are decreasing (Schmidtke, 1995). Also, in the WHO/EURO Multicentre Study on Parasuicide, there is no significant covariation between the unemployment rate and the suicide attempt rate within the various centers (Bille-Brahe et al., 1996). Studies also show that especially the teenage suicide rates are not related to the quality of life (Lester, 1988). However, time series analyses on differenced data from 1911 to 1990 in Norway showed that alcohol consumption and divorce were independently and statistically significantly associated with the male suicide rate, but not with the female suicide rate (Rossow, 1993).

Religious Beliefs and Affiliations

Geographical differences between the European countries are also confounded by differences in religious variables. The various European countries differ with regard to the percentage of the main religions. Previous studies show, for example, significant coavariations between the rates of suicide and of undetermined deaths and the main religious affiliation even within a country. In more Catholic regions, the suicide rates are mostly lower, and the rate of undetermined death higher; whereas the suicide rates are higher in more protestant regions (Bojanovsky, 1979, 1981). One reason for this might be the different religions' reactions with regard to their funeral ceremonies. In some Catholic regions, suicide victims were not buried with religious ceremonies, therefore increasing the probability to hide a suicide. However, the results of the WHO/EURO Multicentre Study on Parasuicide show that this hypothesis today cannot explain any great part of the variances. For example, in Würzburg, Germany, an area with primarily Catholic population, the religious affiliation of the suicide attempters shows no difference from the general population (Schmidtke, Fricke, & Weinacker, 1994).

Attitudes and Legislation

If a behavior is culturally sanctioned, the probability of such behavior is lower. Thus, an important target for the explanation of differences and primary prevention may be local, perhaps also age- and gender-specific cultures of suicidal behavior (Andriolo, 1984; Canetto & Lester, 1995; Draguns, 1994; Leenaars, 1995; Platt, 1989, 1993; Retterstol, 1993). Sociocultural attitudes and the role of elderly people in society have, for example, a significant relevance for the incidence of suicide in the elderly. Their differences in the European countries may, therefore, explain the significant differences among the suicide rates of the elderly (Bron, 1989). Cultural attitudes toward individual suicide methods also play an important role in how often they will be used for suicide (Snowdon, 1978).

General Attitudes

The most striking finding within Europe is the different and changing attitudes toward suicide (Diekstra & Garnefski, 1995). The European countries differ significantly, for example, regarding the number of headlines with suicide themes. There was a significant difference for the year 1981 between the eastern and western countries, with nearly no reports in the eastern countries. With regard to the content, there were also significant differences between the eastern and western countries. Whereas, for example, the rate of "positive" prominent celebrities was highest in Hungary, suicide reports of "negative" celebrities were significantly more frequent in German headlines. Reports containing positive consequences of suicidal behavior were also more frequent in Hungary and Lithuania, whereas negative consequences of suicidal behavior are more often described in German and Austrian headlines.

Some preliminary results for the differences between the United States and Hungary show more prominent names in Hungarian headlines. More American headlines label suicide in a more criminalizing way, whereas the suicidal behavior is portrayed more as tragedy and political protest in the Hungarian headlines. It seems that – on the basis of presented consequences, qualifications, and wordings in the headlines – there are rather accepting attitudes toward suicide in the Hungarian and Lithuanian media. One can hypothesize that these evaluations and the labeling in the media presentations reflect the different attitudes of the several cultures toward suicide. According to the basic research, the portrayal of positive consequences of suicidal behavior increases and the portrayal of negative consequences decreases the possibility of identification and imitation with a suicide model. Therefore, Diekstra and Garnefski (1995) for example, also see one reason for the increase of suicidal behavior among adolescents in the more frequent presentation of suicide models.

Some survey studies also show different attitudes toward suicide behavior. One hypothesis for the explanation of the high suicide rates in the former German Democratic Republic is that different attitudes toward psychological aspects in politics enhance suicidal behavior (Belau, 1991). Swedish adolescents have more liberal attitudes toward suicide than Turkish adolescents. However, Turkish adolescents show greater acceptance for a suicidal peer than Swedish adolescents (Eskin, 1995a). Also the attitudes toward life and death are different (Weiss & Perry, 1975). However, the differences in attitudes are not reflected in suicide notes. A recent comparison between German and U.S. suicide notes revealed no major differences with regard to several aspects (Leenaars et al., 1994).

The cultural characteristics and attitudes of a population may also affect the relevant importance of the various factors involved in suicidal attempts. For example, findings indicate that suppression of personal freedom by parents is a major risk factor for suicidal attempts in Greek female adolescents (Beratis, 1990, 1991).

Legislation

Attitudes toward a behavior are mainly reflected in the legislation with regard to this behavior. Defining a behavior as a medical problem can change both its moral and legal consequences (MacDonald, 1989). Therefore, a further hypothesis is that these differences are mainly caused by the differences in the legislation regarding suicide and assisting suicidal behavior, with more lenient laws, for example, in the Netherlands (Diekstra, 1993) and stricter laws in the southern parts of Europe. In some parts of Europe, first in the early 1960s, suicidal behavior was no longer "illegal" and regarded as "crime" (under the penal code). In Germany, assisting suicidal behavior for nondoctors is generally not forbidden because according to the law assistance cannot be punished if the main behavior (delict) is not punished. However, in Austria, assisting suicide by a nondoctor is illegal. Also, the regulations and contracts of the insurance companies in the various countries differ widely with regard to payments after a suicide. Although all of these laws also reflect cultural differences in attitudes toward suicidal behavior, no study exists that evaluated these differences. However, there are some hypotheses that "normalizing" suicide as a medical option through legalization of assisted suicide may build the groundwork for a society that turns euthanasia into a "cure" for suicidal depression (Hendin, 1995).

Individual Coping Strategies

There are some hypotheses that the various European countries differ with regard to differences of their individuals. They assume differences in the level of intraversion–extraversion, impulsivity, and the coping strategies for stress. For example, in comparison to Turkish adolescents with suicide attempts, a study of Swedish adolescents with suicide attempts found more low positive assertion skills (Eskin, 1995b). Robertson and Cochrane (1976) assume that a change has occurred in the world view of young people, and that this has been responsible for the differential increase in attempted suicide. The elements of this change were seen as an emphasis on the importance of "self-fulfillment"; a belief that society, rather than the individual, should be responsible for providing the means to personal fulfillment; and a resulting tendency to regard social and material deprivations as obstacles to self-fulfillment. It was postulated that individuals who possess these values, and who live in objectively deprived circumstances, would be less willing to tolerate stress than would their older counterparts, who were seen as emphasizing personal fulfillment and personal responsibility. A set of hypotheses derived from this model was tested in a study of 100 male attempted suicides and 100 controls. The findings supported the view that changes of the type suggested have taken place in the consciousness of young people, but these do not seem to relate to the trend in attempted suicide among the young. Therefore, up to now, no convincing study exists showing significant covariations. In contrast, results suggest that probably no clear link between attitudes and actual suicidal behavior at the societal level exists (Kerkhof & Nathawat, 1989), and that the personality correlates of suicidal tendencies are rather similar despite differences in age and cultural background (Irfani, 1978).

PREVENTION STRATEGIES

Perhaps based on different attitudes, the European countries also differ widely with regard to their prevention strategies. Whereas organizations like the Samaritans were founded relatively early in the United Kingdom (the primary goal of these organizations is suicide prevention), no such organizations were present until 1989 in the eastern countries. Also, the date of foundation of the different national suicide prevention organizations differs widely: Austria has one of the first (international) organizations—perhaps due to its high suicide rate—and Switzerland funded such an organization relatively late. In some countries, even the various local organizations do not share the same names (i.e., in Germany). The various nations also differ with regard to national suicide prevention programs (e.g., in Finland, Sweden) and funds for such programs, like in Germany. However, this partially depends on the structure of the different countries and on their constitution. In recent years the European Union (EU) sponsored some research on suicidal behavior (i.e., parts of the WHO/EURO Multicentre Study on Parasuicide) and a survey on suicide prevention programs and organizations in the EU.

CONCLUSION

The differences between the various European countries with regard to suicide and suicide attempt rates are enormous. Despite the fact that such differences exist, variations in ascertainment procedures and methodological artifacts due to different age structures and percentages of immigrants cannot explain the major part of these variances. Also, economic hypotheses cannot explain these differences. To date, besides some ethnic hypotheses, the most convincing hypotheses are those based on different attitudes toward suicidal behavior.

REFERENCES

Andriolo, K. R. (1984). Selbstmord als Krise der Gemeinschaft—Zur gesellschaftlichen Bewertung der Selbsttötung im transkulturellen Vergleich. *Psychosozial, 23*, 56–67.

Belau, D. (1991). Interpretation der Selbsttötung auf dem Hintergrund der DDR-Kultur. *Suizidprophylaxe, 18*, 271–285.

Beratis, S. (1990). Factors associated with adolescent suicidal attempts in Greece. *Psychopathology, 23*, 161–168.

Beratis, S. (1991). Suicide attempts and suicides in Greek adolescents. In D. Papadatou & C. papadatos (Eds.), *Children and death* (pp. 77–84). (Series in Death Education, Aging, and Health Care). New York: Hemisphere.

Bille-Brahe, U., Kerkhof, A. DeLeo, D., et al. (1996). A repetition prediction study on European parasuicide populations. Part II of the WHO/EURO Multicentre Study on Parasuicide in cooperation with the EC concerted action on attempted suicide. *Crisis, 17*, 22–31.

Bojanovsky, J. (1979). Leben Protestanten Länger? *Medizin, Mensch, Gesellschaft, 4*, 120–123.

Bojanovsky, J. (1981). Religion und Lebenserwartung. *Lebensversicherungsmedizin, 33*, 141–142.

Bron, B. (1989). Suizidalitat im Alter. *Fortschritte der Medizin, 107*, 266–270.

Canetto, S. S., & Lester, D. (1995). Gender and the primary prevention of suicide mortality. *Suicide and Life-Threatening Behavior, 25*, 58–69.

Connolly, J. F., & Cullen, A. U. (1995). Underreporting of suicide in an Irish county. *Crisis, 16*, 34–38.

DeLeo, D., Carollo, G., Dello Buono, M. Conforti, D., & Mastinu, A. (1995). Epidemiology of suicide in the elderly population of Italy: 1958–1988. Archives of Suicide Research, I, 3–17.

Diekstra, R. F. W. (1993). Assisted suicide and euthanasia: Experiences from The Netherlands. *Annals of Medicine, 25*, 5–9.

Diekstra, R. F. W. (1996). The epidemiology of suicide and parasuicide. *Archives of Suicide Research, 2*, 1–29.

Diekstra, R. F. W., & Garnefski, N. (1995). On the nature, magnitude, and causality of suicidal behaviors: An international perspective. *Suicide and Life-Threatening Behavior, 25*, 36–57.

Draguns, J. G. (1994). Pathological and clinical aspects. In L. Loeb Adler & U. P. Gielen (Eds.), *Cross-cultural topics in psychology* (pp. 165-177). Westport, CT: Praeger Publishers/Greenwood.

Eskin, M. (1995a). Adolescents' attitudes toward suicide, and a suicidal peer: A comparison between Swedish and Turkish high school students. *Scandinavian Journal of Psychology, 36*, 201-207.

Eskin, M. (1995b). Suicidal behavior as related to social support and assertiveness among Swedish and Turkish high school students: A cross-cultural investigation. *Journal of Clinical Psychology, 51*, 158-172.

Gulbinat, W. (1996). The epidemiology of suicide in old age. *Archives of Suicide Research, 2*, 31-42.

Hendin, H. (1995). Assisted suicide, euthanasia, and suicide prevention: The implications of the Dutch experience. *Suicide and Life-Threatening Behavior, 25*, 193-204.

Irfani, S. (1978). Personality correlates of suicidal tendency among Iranian and Turkish students. *Journal of Psychology, 99*, 151-153.

Kerkhof, A., & Nathawat, S. S. (1989). Suicidal behavior and attitudes towards suicide among students in India and the Netherlands: A cross-cultural comparison. In R. F. W. Diekstra, R. Maris, S. Platt, A. Schmidtke, & G. Sonneck (Eds.), *Suicide and its prevention: The role of attitude and imitation* (pp. 144-159) (Advances in Suicidology, Vol. 1). Leiden: Brill.

Leenaars, A. (1995). Suicide. In H. Wass & R. A. Neimeyer (Eds.), *Dying: Facing the facts* (3rd ed.) (pp. 347-383) (Series in Death Education, Aging, and Health Care). Philadelphia: Taylor & Francis.

Leenaars, A., Lester, D., Wenckstern, -S. Heim, N. (1994). Suizid-Abschiedsbriefe – Ein Vergleich deutscher und amerikanischer Abschiedsbriefe von Suizidenten. *Suizidprophylaxe, 21*, 99-101.

Lester, D. (1972). *Why people kill themselves.* Springfield, IL: C. C. Thomas.

Lester, D. (1982). The distribution of sex and age among completed suicides: A cross-national study. *International Journal of Social Psychiatry, 28*, 256-260.

Lester, D. (1988). Youth suicide: A cross-cultural perspective. *Adolescence, 23*, 955-958.

MacDonald, M. (1989). The medicalization of suicide in England: Laymen, physicians, and cultural change, 1500-1870. *Milbank Quarterly, 67*(Suppl. 1), 69-91.

Milcinski, L., & Mrevlje, G. (1990). Epidemiologija samoubistva u Jugoslaviji-metodoloska pitanja. *Medicinski Pregled, 43*, 453-456.

Moksony, F. (1995). The age pattern of suicide in Hungary. *Archives of Suicide Research, 1*, 217-222.

Morselli, H. (1881). *Der Selbstmord.* Leipzig: Brockhaus.

Mösler, T. A., Pontzen, W., & Rummler, W. (1990). The relationship between suicidal acts and unemployment. In G. Ferrari, M. Bellini, & P. Crepet (Eds.), *Suicidal behavior and risk factors.* Bologna: Monduzzi.

Petronis, K. R., Samuels, J. F., Moscicki, E. K., & Anthony, J. C. (1990). An epidemiologic investigation of potential risk factors for suicide attempts. *Social Psychiatry and Psychiatric Epidemiology, 25*, 193-199.

Platt, S. (1986). Parasuicide and unemployment. *British Journal of Psychiatry, 149*, 401-405.

Platt, S. (1989). A subculture of parasuicide? In R. F. W. Diekstra, R. Maris, S. Platt, A., Schmidtke, & G. Sonneck (Eds.), *Suicide and its prevention: The role of attitude and imitation* (pp. 108-143) (Advances in Suicidology, Vol. 1). Leiden: Brill.

Platt, S. (1993). Is there a suicidal subculture? *Crisis.*

Platt, S., Bille-Brahe, U., Kerkhof, A., Schmidtke, A., et al. (1992). Parasuicide in Europe: The WHO/EURO Multicentre Study on Parasuicide. I. Introduction and preliminary analysis for 1989. *Acta Psychiatrica Scandinavica, 85*, 97-104.

Platt, S., & Kreitman, N. (1985). Is unemployment a cause of parasuicide? *British Medical Journal, 290*, 161.

Retterstol, N. (1993). *Suicide: A European perspective.* Cambridge: The University Press.

Robertson, A., & Cochrane, R.(1976). Attempted suicide and cultural change: An empirical investigation. *Human Relations, 29*, 863-883.

Rossow, I. (1993). Suicide, alcohol, and divorce: Aspects of gender and family integration. *Addiction, 88*, 1659-1665.

Rygnestad, T., & Hauge, L. (1991). Epidemiological, social and psychiatric aspects in self-poisoned patients. A prospective comparative study from Trondheim, Norway between 1978 and 1987. *Social Psychiatry and Psychiatric Epidemiology, 26*, 53-62.

Sainsbury, P. (1983). Validity and reliability of trends in suicide statistics. *Health Statistics Quarterly, 36*, 339-348.

Sainsbury, P., & Barraclough, B. M. (1968). Differences between suicide rates. *Nature, 220*, 1252.

Schmidtke, A. (1989). *WHO (Euro) Multicentre Study of Parasuicide.* Working paper for the WHO Consultation on Strategies for Reducing Suicidal Behaviour in the European Region, Szeged, Hungary, ICP/PSF 024/18.

Schmidtke, A. (1995). Suizid- und Suizidversuchsraten in Deutschland. In M. Wolfersdorf & W. Kaschka, (Hrsg.), *Suizidalität – Die biologische Dimension* (pp. 17-32). Heidelberg: Springer, 17-32.

Schmidtke, A., Bille-Brahe, U., DeLeo, D., Kerkhof, A., Bjerke, T., Crepet, P., Haring, C., Hawton, K., Lönnqvist, J., Michel, K., Pommereau, X., Querejeta, I., Phillippe, I., Salander-Renberg, E., Temesváry, B., Wasserman, D., Weinacker, B., & Sampaio-Faria, J. (1995). *Suicide and suicide attempt rates in Europe, 1989-1993.* Paper presented at the XVIII International IASP Congress, Venice (Abstract Book: 31).

Schmidtke, A., Bille-Brahe, U., DeLeo, D., Kerkhof, A., Bjerke, T., Crepet, P., Haring, C., Hawton, K., Lönnqvist, J., Michel, K., Pommereau, X., Querejeta, J., Phillippe, I., Salander-Renberg, E., Temesváry, B., Wasserman, D., Fricke, S., Weinacker, B., & Sampaio-Faria, J. (1996, in press). Attempted suicide in Europe: Rates, trends, and sociodemographic characteristics of suicide attempters, 1989-1992. Results of the WHO/EURO Multicentre Study on Parasuicide. *Acta Psychiatrica Scandinavica.*

Schmidtke, A., Bille-Brahe, U., Kerkhof, A., DeLeo, D., Platt, S., Sampaio-Faria, J., Henderson, J., &

Pototzky, W. (1993). The WHO/EURO Multicentre Project on Parasuicide–State of the art. *Italian Journal of Suicidology, 3,* 83-95.

Schmidtke, A., Fricke, S., & Weinacker, B. (1994). The epidemiology of attempted suicide in the Würzburg area, Germany 1989-1992. In A. J. F. M. Kerkhof, A. Schmidtke, U. Bille-Brahe, D. DeLeo, & J. Lönnqvist, (Eds.), *Attempted suicide in Europe* (pp. 159-174). Leiden: DSWO Press.

Schmidtke, A., Häfner, H., Möller, H. J., Wedler, H., & Böhme, K. (1988). Häufigkeiten und Trends von Suizidversuchen in der Bundesrepublik Deutschland: Eine methodische Studie. *Öffentliches Gesundheitswesen, 50,* 272-277.

Schmidtke, A., & Weinacker, B. (1991). Covariation of suicides and undetermined deaths among elderly persons: A methodological study. *Crisis, 12,* 44-58.

Schmidtke, A., & Weinacker, B. (1993). Do the official suicide rates among older persons represent the true magnitude of the problem? In Böhme, K., Freytag, R., Wächtler, C., & Wedler, H. (Eds.), *Suicidal behavior–The state of the art* (pp. 113-117). Regensburg: Roderer.

Snowdon, J. (1978). Suicide in Australia-A comparison with suicide in England and Wales. *Australian and New Zealand Journal of Psychiatry, 13,* 301-307.

Snyder, M. L. (1994). Methods of suicide used by Irish and Japanese samples: A cross-cultural study from 1964 to 1979. *Psychological Reports, 74,* 127-130.

Värnik, A., & Wassermann, D. (1992). Suicide in the former Soviet republics. *Acta Psychiatrica Scandinavica, 86,* 76-78.

Wedel, H. (1992). *Mortality data in the states around the Baltic.* Paper presented at the Symposium Epidemiology Around the Baltic Sea, Stockholm, Royal Medical Society.

Weiss, J. M., & Perry, M. E. (1975). Transcultural attitudes toward homocide and suicide. *Suicide, 5,* 223-227.

WHO. (1982). *Changing patterns of suicide behaviour.* Copenhagen: WHO, Regional Office for Europe.

WHO. (1995). *World Health Statistics Annual 1994.* Geneva: Author.

WHO. (1992). *Health-for-all targets. The health policy for Europe* Summary of the updated edition, September 1991. Copenhagen: Author (EUR ICP/HSC 013).

Winkler, W. F. (1960). Über den Wandel in Häufigkeit, Bedingungen und Beurteilung des Suicids in der Nachkriegszeit. *Der Öffentliche Gesundheitsdienst, 22,* 135-145.

14
Culture and Suicide: From a Japanese Psychiatrist's Perspective

Yoshitomo Takahashi, MD

There have been numerous papers focusing on culture and suicide, but it seems that they have often emphasized cultural differences excessively, thus running the risk of increasing prejudice toward different cultures and reinforcing overgeneralizations. From my albeit limited knowledge and experience, it appears that there are more similarities than differences in suicide among various cultures. Most cases of suicide reflect complex human factors that are found universally among cultures. Despite the fact that some cultural differences in suicide admittedly exist in different societies and that these are important, they cannot explain every aspect of suicide. This article explains how I, as a Japanese psychiatrist, diagnose and treat suicidal patients against the backgrounds of Japanese culture by presenting my way of thinking in daily practice in order to show similarities and differences that exist in Japanese suicide, treatment, and prevention.

Various renowned scholars have stated that Japanese show different attitude toward suicide from the rest of the world. Ruth Benedict, American anthropologist, wrote in her classical work *The Chrysanthemum and the Sword* (1974):

> The most extreme aggressive action a modern Japanese takes against himself is suicide. Suicide, properly done, will, according to their tenets, clear his name and reinstate his memory. American condemnation of suicide makes self-destruction only a desperate submission to despair, but the Japanese respect for it allows it to be an honorable and purposeful act. In certain situations it is the most honorable course to take in *giri* to one's name. (p. 166)

Mamoru Iga (1993), a sociologist, mentioned: "In Japan, suicide has traditionally been an accepted, if not welcomed, way of solving a serious problem" (p. 301).

Some also have shown concern about the high suicide rate of Japanese young people. Edwin O. Reischauer, who was an American ambassador to Japan, professor of Harvard University, and world-renowned Japanologist, stated: "The relatively high suicide rates for youth may be in part attributable to the 'examination hell' " (Reischauer & Jansen, 1995, p. 194). Richard Seiden (1966) also mentioned, in referring to the Japanese situation regarding academic pressure and suicide: "There are tremendous pressures to attend college, and those students who fail to gain entrance frequently turn to suicide as a solution to their dilemmas" (p. 394).

However, these opinions do not necessarily reflect the actual situation of suicide in Japan. It is true that Japan once showed a high suicide rate, in the 1950s, but its suicide rate has been decreasing gradually but steadily. The suicide rate in Japan is not unusually high compared to other nations. In 1993 there were 21,679 suicides in Japan, which makes the suicide rate about 17 per 100,000 population. This places it in the middle of the rates for some European countries. Therefore, the widely believed view that "suicide is extremely common in Japan" is myth, probably due to overemphasis of *hara-kiri* (self-disembowelment by feudal warriors),

Yoshitomo Takahashi, MD, is with the Department of Psychopathology, Tokyo Institute of Psychiatry, Kamikitazawa, Setagaya-ku, Tokyo 156, Japan. Fax: 81-3-3329-8035; E-mail: fred@prit.go.jp

Suicide and Life-Threatening Behavior, Vol. 27(1), Spring 1997

kamikaze pilots, and suicides of novelists such as Osamu Dazai, Yukio Mishima, Yasunari Kawabata, et al. The suicide rate of Japanese for 15 to 24-year-olds is actually lower than that of the United States.

When Japanese suicide is discussed, too much attention is often paid to cultural differences. In fact it should be stressed that there are more similarities than differences in suicide between different cultures. Suicidal Japanese have just as many "risk factors" for suicide as those in other countries, including psychiatric disorders, prior suicide attempts, lack of social support systems, male preponderance, older age, various kinds of loss, family history of suicide, and accident proneness.

There have been numerous papers focusing on culture and suicide. However, upon reading such papers, I have noticed that they often place excessive emphasis on cultural differences, thus running the risk of increasing prejudice toward different cultures and reinforcing overgeneralizations. From my admittedly limited knowledge and experience, it seems that more similarities than differences in suicide exist in various cultures, and that previous papers have underestimated this perspective and have emphasized only the differences.

In writing this article, I wish to make a conscious effort to avoid strengthening any fixed idea the reader may have about Japanese suicide. In fact, I have often asked myself whether uniquely "Japanese" suicide really exists. I consider that most cases of suicide reflect complex human factors that are found universally among cultures. Although cultural differences in suicide admittedly exist in different societies and are important, I do not believe that they can explain every aspect of suicide.

In this article, instead of reviewing previous studies on culture and suicide, I will give an outline of how, as a Japanese psychiatrist, I diagnose and treat suicidal patients against the backgrounds of Japanese culture by explaining my way of thinking, which I hope will show the reader the similarities and differences that exist in Japanese suicide, treatment, and prevention.

GENERAL ATTITUDE TOWARD SUICIDE IN JAPAN

Before discussing the main theme, I would like to explain briefly the attitude of Japanese people toward suicide in general. Although it has been suggested that attitudes toward suicide vary among cultures, there have been few comparative studies between Japan and other countries based on the same methodology. Domino and Takahashi (1991) studied attitudes toward suicide in Japan and the United States using the Suicide Opinion Questionnaire, and the findings indicated that the Japanese were more likely to think that suicide is not always an abnormal form of behavior, and that it might be permissible in certain situations. In contrast, the Americans were more likely to think that suicide is usually a result of some psychiatric problem in which aggression is directed toward the self, and that suicide should be prevented. Because the sample size in this study was limited, the findings should not be overgeneralized, although the study was meaningful because it utilized the same data base in both countries. The results suggest that, in a culture where suicide may be permissible, social factors may need to be taken into consideration.

It is a fact that Japan is popularly held to be a country in which suicide is permissible to some extent. It is often reported to the world that the Japanese regard suicide as an honorable way to take responsibility, similar to *hara-kiri,* the traditional form of suicide committed by warriors in the feudal era.

However, in contemporary Japanese society, suicidal people often consider that death is the only way of resolving a desperate situation, being neither an honorable form of behavior nor a tradition condoned by society. In fact, there is a strong stigma against suicide and intense prejudice toward the mental disorders related to it, and this makes ordinary Japanese individuals reluctant to seek help from mental health professionals. They fear that they might be ostracized if they are diagnosed as suffering from psychiatric disorder, which is a shame for them and their families. (Intense social stigma toward suicide is one of the reasons why there have been few biological researches or psychological autopsy studies on suicide in Japan.)

If suicide does occur, those left behind have to bear a lifelong stigma that a family member took his or her own life. Unlike Americans, Japanese do not offer spontaneous help to the bereaved of suicide victims, and conversely, the latter also do not accept help offered from people outside the family. It is generally believed that people should behave as if nothing has happened, never touching upon the subject, and that time is the only panacea for healing their wound.

ASPECTS OF CAUTION IN THE TREATMENT OF SUICIDAL JAPANESE PATIENTS

Let us assume a situation in which a patient with a suicidal problem visits a psychiatric clinic. The patient and the psychotherapist are both Japanese. The consultation room is located in the outpatient department of psychiatry at a general hospital.

The opening situation related to the therapy itself may seem different from that to which the American reader is accustomed. As stated already, the average Japanese attitude is not to seek psychiatric help directly and openly, or to speak about suicide frankly. Because of the strong social stigma toward psychiatric disorders in Japanese society, patients are usually afraid of coming to a psychiatric clinic of their own free will and are often brought reluctantly or forced to attend by family members.

Therefore, psychiatrists need to adopt certain tactics to alleviate patients' anxiety at the first encounter. Not all Japanese psychiatrists use the same tactics; I will describe the style that I employ, and many of my colleagues behave in a similar way.

My hair is cut short and combed, and I have neither a mustache nor a beard. I wear a starched white shirt and a conservative tie. My eyeglasses are also ordinary ones. In addition, when at the hospital, I wear a white gown. In fact, most Japanese psychiatrists look like physicians of internal medicine. The consultation room is very quiet, neat, and comfortable in order for patients to speak with ease, although it looks like a room in a department of internal medicine. All this effort is aimed at reducing the anxiety of the patient, who has often been taken by others to the hospital against his or her will. In short, the average Japanese psychiatrist tries to project an image corresponding more closely to the conventional image of a physician that patients have. I try not to emphasize my own uniqueness to the patient at the beginning, because I know that my own personality characteristics will appear gradually as the long-term psychotherapy advances.

In cases where the family have taken a patient to the psychiatric clinic, I invite them to enter the consultation room together and ask them whether (1) the patient would first like to speak to me alone, (2) the family would first like to speak to me alone, or (3) both the patient and family members would like to stay and speak together. Some patients are afraid that the family and I will decide to carry out some undesirable treatment without their consent; some ask the family to explain their problem first because they think that the problem is too complicated for them to explain alone; and some wish to explain by themselves but are too anxious, and wish the family to stay with them during the first examination.

My first target of psychotherapy is to establish a rapport with the patient (Takahashi, 1989), as other clinicians have pointed out (Hendren, 1990; Jacobs, 1989; Mintz, 1988; Shneidman, 1985). Sometimes it is difficult to open up to each other among Japanese, and an awkward silence may continue for an extended period. This is especially the case at the first encounter with a suicidal patient, but I let this silence continue for some time. Generally speaking, in comparison with Americans, Japanese are not very good at articulating their opinions from the beginning.

It is widely accepted in North America that talking about suicide openly promotes understanding and can greatly decrease the immediate distress of a suicidal person. Asking a patient directly if he or she is considering suicide is encouraged: If the person is feeling suicidal, it can come as a great relief to see that someone else has some idea of how he or she feels.

Basically, I agree with this principle, but for Japanese patients the situation seems more complicated. Although helping the patient to share the despair with the therapist is important, with Japanese patients it is sometimes very difficult to bring the topic of suicide into the open. Therefore, I do not think that it is a good strategy to start asking Japanese patients "Have you ever thought about committing suicide?" or "Have you attempted suicide before?" directly within minutes after starting the first session.

When it is apparent to the patient that the therapist has a sincere and honest desire to alleviate the patient's overwhelming distress, the patient's anxiety will gradually abate. This is often time consuming and seems inefficient, but I consider it important to wait for the patient to gradually open his mind. In a Japanese cultural context, it is tacitly accepted that a patient's silence does not necessarily mean that he or she has nothing to say, and that certain kinds of silence can convey depth of thought.

I need to get some idea of the kinds of problems the patient has had in the past that might have led to suicidal ideation or behavior. I also need to examine how severe the patient's despair is, how the future is accepted, what kinds of hopes and expectations are held for the future, how the relationship between the world and the person is regarded, how the patient values him/herself in the world, and the reactions to previous problematic situations (Takahashi, 1993b). I, then, have to sort out the patient's problems, feed them back to verify whether I have understood them correctly, and show the patient that I am sympathetic by saying things like "You have had numerous difficult problems." After a rapport has been established with the patient, he or she will often begin to speak about the suicidal ideation voluntarily.

Finally, I will inquire directly about suicidal intent, method of suicide, its lethality, plans to repeat suicidal behavior, and whether this is intended to act as a message to specific individuals. I think that, in general, Japanese psychotherapists do spend more time than American therapists establishing a rapport with patients before asking them directly about suicide.

Needless to say, I examine the patient for other risk factors, such as psychiatric disorder and its severity, treatment, prior history of suicide attempts, various kinds of loss, lack of support systems, accident proneness, family history of suicide, and child abuse (Takahashi, 1992). Detailed information on these points has to be collected. However, it is rare to be able to collect all the necessary information at the first session and I spend several sessions for this purpose, because it has high priority. The important point here once again is to balance the establishment of a rapport with the collection of the necessary data for the evaluation of suicide risk.

If possible, I request as many members of the patient's family as possible to come to the clinic so that I can observe directly the interaction of all the members including the patient. This principle is what I learned from Joseph Richman's (1986) *Family Therapy for Suicidal People.* The process of introducing the family members to therapy also shows an aspect of informed consent and emphasizes that the cooperation of the family is indispensable for successful treatment. I always explain repeatedly to the family members that therapeutic exchanges between the patient and myself alone are not enough for overcoming the suicidal crisis, and that family members should also cooperate.

In addition, because of their self-blame or mechanism of denial, the family members often try to underestimate the patient's problem. I take time to explain that suicide risk is not a mere threat but a genuine cry for help from the patient. I regard this process of family participation in the therapy as meaningful, especially for the suicidal patient. The process of psychotherapy will gradually reveal that the patient's psychopathology is not merely a problem for that individual but a reflection of the psychopathology that all the family members have.

Although it is often pointed out that Japanese family structures have been changing recently, the family bond is still strong in Japan, and therefore perspectives of family involvement in therapy for the suicidal patient are all the more important. If the family members are asked for cooperation, they are usually willing to offer help, even though their attitude is initially pathological, to become part of a therapeutic alliance. Otherwise, if they know later that a patient has sought psychotherapy without telling other family members, they will often demand that the patient should terminate the therapy because of social stigma or the mechanism of denial.

From a practical viewpoint, I also ask family members to remove from the home any potentially lethal items that could be used for suicide (often to manage medication, if necessary) and to become key persons who can offer first intervention measures to the patient if necessary.

If a patient seeks psychiatric help by him/herself without mentioning it to the family and the suicide risk is considered very high, I explain to the patient why family contact is necessary, obtain consent, contact the family members, and ask them to participate in the therapy.

As for the issue of a contract against suicide, few Japanese psychotherapists will ask a patient for a written contract stating that he or she will never commit suicide before seeking help when faced with a serious situation. Instead, before closing the first session, I ask the patient verbally to promise to contact me if he or she is doubtful about controlling the suicidal impulses. Although a contract against suicide, either verbal or written, is considered to have no legal basis in Japan, I try to gauge the patient's suicide risk by raising this topic and evaluating the degree of willingness (or unwillingness) to participate in a therapeutic alliance. It is very important for me to see how the patient responds to this request after establishing some degree of rapport and evaluating suicide risk using a formal approach. As Simon (1987) has mentioned, a contract against suicide may be useful in certain instances by reaffirming the therapeutic alliance, but its limitations should be clearly understood. It goes without saying that I also indicate to the patient how I can be contacted or other staff can be reached on a 24-hour basis if he or she is in a critical situation. Concrete arrangements should also be made for the next appointment by discussion with the patient.

The above procedures are those employed for the first session with the suicidal patient. Because it is rare that the suicidal crisis will be averted immediately, and because characteristically such crises tend to recur, I take precautionary measures against future suicidal crises and introduce the patient to long-term psychotherapy. It is especially important to find a treatment setting that allows a close relationship between outpatient therapy and an inpatient therapy.

Along with intensive psychopharmacological therapy for the psychiatric disorders that underlie the suicidal crisis, psychotherapy is extremely important for suicidal patients. Although, due to lack of space I am unable to give a detailed description here, an efficient form of intervention is cognitive behavioral therapy focusing on the patient's dysfunctional behavior pattern in daily life (Beck, 1976; Freeman, Pretzer, Fleming, & Simon, 1990; Freeman, & Reinecke, 1993). I believe that cognitive behavioral therapy is valuable for suicidal Japanese patients because it gives both patients and therapists a common language for discussing problems. (Cognitive therapy has been gradually gaining ground in Japan recently, although it is still not used very widely by Japanese mental health professionals. The reader should bear in mind that the above description of cognitive behavioral therapy for suicidal Japanese patients is limited only to my own personal style of psychotherapy.)

SUICIDE RISK OVER THE LIFE CYCLE

At this point, it is probably useful to briefly discuss suicide risk over the life cycle in a Japanese cultural context. In order to understand the psychology of a patient (especially one contemplating suicide) in a given culture, it is necessary to decipher the different idiomatic forms of distress inherent to that culture. Here, I will refer specifically to the adolescent patient, the young mother, the middle-aged man, and the elderly patient in relation to problems faced by Japanese society. Once again, the relationship between the self and others (family, organization, society, etc.) is the key concept for understanding the psychology of suicide over the life cycle.

The Adolescent Patient

The family's problems have a great influence on the suicidal adolescent. Therefore, I try to understand whether the patient's symptoms arise only from him/herself or from the whole family's psychopathology.

It has often been pointed out that entrance examinations for prestigious universities in Japan are so difficult that success or failure can decide one's whole life. Fortunately, the "examination hell" is not as severe as it used to be, and society is beginning to recognize various human values. However, academic performance still remains a very important issue for the Japanese adolescent.

I carefully try to determine whether the adolescent patient has been overwhelmed by family pressure in such a social atmosphere and forced into a corner by the characteristic adolescent "black or white," "all or none" dichotomous way of thinking.

There are some adolescents who seem well adjusted superficially and show superb academic performance, but desperately try to overreach their ability in order to obtain the family's attention and love. Some of these adolescents have a deep-seated lack of confidence in their ability and are terrified of failure. Once such a long-dreaded failure actually occurs, even though it might be regarded as a trivial one by other people, the adolescent regards it as a monumental blunder that will have a lifelong effect. The adolescent may even feel that the meaning of life itself has been lost.

For adolescent patients, it is thus more important to appreciate how they regard failure subjectively than to attach a merely objective meaning to the failure. A failure considered by adults to be a minor one and easy to overcome, might seem a "life or death" problem to a vulnerable adolescent. I try to understand the personality characteristics of adolescence and how such patients regard a recently experienced failure.

The Young Mother

Although Japanese social structures have been changing gradually, women, once they get married, are still expected to play a role as housewives in charge of the family and mothers to take care of the children. When such women become depressed for some reason and suicidal, it is necessary to determine whether aggression might be directed not only toward themselves but also toward their children, and if necessary, to ask other family members (sometimes their parents' family) for help.

The Japanese word *shinju* means literally "oneness of mind" (Inamura, 1977; Ohara, 1963; Takahashi, 1993a). It was originally used to mean a lovers' suicide pact based on a mutual agreement, but now it has become used more widely to mean a murder–suicide complex. If a mother, usually in her 20s or 30s, kills her small children and then commits suicide, this act is called *boshi* (mother–child)-*shinju*. The children that are most often the victims of *boshi-shinju* are of preschool age. Needless to say, as children cannot consent to suicide, this is strictly murder–suicide. Emotionally, however, Japanese regard this as extended suicide in which the mother does not kill unrelated individuals but destroys "part of herself." The border between the mother and her children is very obscure, and even a delusional symbiotic bond is sometimes observed. Society is largely sympathetic to such a mother who has been unable to find any other way of solving her problems, and does not criticize her behavior. Conversely, the attitude towards a mother who has killed only herself and left her children alive may be distinctly unsympathetic.

In Japan, the mother–child bond and the mother's dedication to the child are emphasized; paradoxically, it is this very bond that causes *boshi-shinju*. According to Japanese logic, a suicidal mother cannot bear to leave her children to survive alone; she would rather kill them because she believes that nobody in the world would take care of them, and that they would be better off dying with her.

Therefore, when a woman with small children becomes depressed and suicidal, I try my utmost to overcome not only the patient's suicidal crisis but also the possible involvement of children.

Besides the risk of *shinju*, it goes without saying that I also make a careful check for various forms of psychopathology in the children because they have a depressed and suicidal mother.

The Middle-Aged Man

When I was a medical student, I was very impressed with an American textbook of psychiatry. The textbook described how to evaluate social adjustment in a given individual. It emphasized the evaluation of various factors including job performance, family life (role as a parent or spouse, etc.), relationship with acquaintances, religious beliefs, contribution to society, and hobbies. This was about 20 years ago when Japanese society was still in a period of rapid economic growth, and when the ideal image of a middle-aged Japanese man was one who sacrificed his life entirely for work and his company, did not take leave, and did not mind having little time to spend with his family.

Unfortunately, Japanese society has not changed substantially since then, and selfless dedication to work and company is still highly valued, especially for middle-aged men. When treating patients of this generation, I pay special attention to the type who identify too intensely with work commitments as being at risk of suicide.

Society often places special significance on *inseki-jisatsu*, which usually means a middle-aged man's suicide in order to take responsibility (Fuse, 1985). Failure at work may trigger such a suicide. Even if it was not particularly the victim's fault, the mere occurrence of some scandal may make him feel responsible. De Vos (1962) called this "role narcissism" or "intense identification of one's self with one's professional self." Role narcissism compels an individual toward suicide when a serious error in role performance has been made by the individual or by another for whom the subject is responsible. A suicide committed out of guilt for having caused trouble to others through a failure in role performance combines intropunitive communication (apology) with role commitment. Not only a committed error but also an anticipated error or failure may induce suicidal anxiety.

In addition, although lifetime employment has been maintained in Japan since the end of World War II, no organization can be immune to drastic restructuring under the current harsh economic conditions. For a middle-aged man who has sacrificed everything for the enterprise, sudden dismissal from the company to which he has identified himself or bankruptcy of the organization might easily trigger a suicidal crisis. In addition to what Maltsberger (1986) pointed out as the suicide risk of a person who can find his value of life only at work, we need to consider the social value attached to work in Japanese society.

The Elderly Patient

The suicide rate among the elderly is much higher than that of any other generation in Japan (Takahashi, 1995; Takahashi et al., 1995). Although individuals aged 65 and over accounted for 14% of the total population in 1993, suicides in this age group accounted for 25% of all suicides.

In relation to the previous section, a man who has devoted himself to work, reached the age of retirement and left the workplace may face a critical situation. It is a serious challenge for Japanese men to readjust themselves to their new stage of life after retirement.

A further problem they face is life with their wives again. As soon as they retire, some men have to face divorce request from wives who feel that they have endured an unacceptable situation for many years and cannot face looking after husbands who are unable to perform domestic tasks for themselves.

Elderly Japanese in particular have strong resistance against consulting psychiatrists and tend to put off asking for a consultation. Generally, when Asians develop depression, they tend to complain of various physical symptoms, and this is much more evident in elderly patients. Compared with other generations, the depressive symptoms of the elderly tend to be atypical. They are likely to develop ill-defined physical symptoms and to consult primary care physicians rather than mental health professionals. Despite repeated examinations, such patients are not diagnosed properly at an early stage and thus are at risk of suicide before they receive proper psychiatric treatment.

I often advise primary care physicians to consider the possibility of depression and refer for psychiatric consultation elderly patients who persistently complain of physical symptoms for which no organic causes can be found by repeated physical examinations. In addition, when such patients come to me for treatment, I initially accept the physical complaints as they are and start the session by examining the physical conditions in detail before commencing psychiatric examination for diagnosis. A further factor that has to be carefully considered is the fear of the Japanese elderly patients of becoming a psychological/financial burden to their families.

CONCLUSION

The issues mentioned here are some of the things I have to consider when I see suicidal Japanese patient. Although I have not been able to explain the long process of psychotherapy in detail, I hope that I have been able to convey some of the features that characterize my clinical approach. My personal perspective is that, although some differences in suicide do exist among various cultures, most aspects of suicide do not show great cross-cultural variations. Suicide is a multifactorial phenomenon involving complex human factors, of which cultural differences represent only a small part.

REFERENCES

Beck, A. T. (1976). *Cognitive therapy and the emotional disorders.* New York: International Universities Press.

Benedict, R. (1974). *The chrysanthemum and the sword.* Tokyo: Charles E. Tuttle.

De Vos, G. A. (1962). Suicide in cross-cultural perspective. In H. L. P. Resnik (Ed.), *Suicidal behavior: Diagnosis and management* (pp. 235–245). Boston: Little, Brown.

Domino, J., & Takahashi, Y. (1991). Attitudes towards suicide in Japanese and American medical students. *Suicide and Life-Threatening Behavior, 21,* 345–359.

Freeman, A., Pretzer, J., Fleming, B., & Simon, K. M. (1990). *Clinical application of cognitive therapy.* New York: Plenum Press.

Freeman, A., & Reinecke, M. A. (1993). *Cognitive therapy of suicidal behavior: A manual for treatment.* New York: Springer.

Fuse, T. (1985). *Suicide and culture.* Tokyo: Shinchosha (in Japanese).

Hendren, R. L. (1990). Assessment and interviewing strategies for suicidal patients over the life cycle. In S. J. Blumenthal & D. J. Kupfer (Eds.), *Suicide over the life cycle: Risk factors, assessment, and treatment of suicidal patients* (pp. 235-252). Washington, DC: American Psychiatric Press.

Iga, M. (1993). Japanese suicide. In A. A. Leenaars (Ed.), *Suicidology: Essays in honor of Edwin S. Shneidman* (pp. 301-323). Northvale NJ: Jason Aronson.

Inamura, H. (1977). *Suicidology.* Tokyo: University of Tokyo Press (in Japanese).

Jacobs, D. (1989). Psychotherapy with suicidal patients: The empathic method. In D. Jacobs & H. N. Brown (Eds.), *Suicide: Understanding and responding* (pp. 329-342). Madison, WI: International Universities Press.

Maltsberger, J. T. (1986). *Suicide risk: The formulation of clinical judgment.* New York: New York University Press.

Mintz, R. S. (1988). Psychotherapy of the depressed suicidal patient. In S. Lesse (Ed.), *What we know about suicidal behavior and how to treat it* (pp. 241-281). Northvale NJ: Jason Aronson.

Ohara, K. (1963). Characteristics of suicide in Japan: Especially on parent-child double suicide. *American Journal of Psychiatry, 120,* 382-385.

Reischauer, E. O., & Jansen, M. B. (1995). *The Japanese today: Change and continuity.* Cambridge: Harvard University Press.

Richman, J. (1986). *Family therapy for suicidal people.* New York: Springer.

Seiden, R. (1966). Campus tragedy: A study of student suicide. *Journal of Abnormal Psychology, 71,* 389-399.

Shneidman, E. S. (1985). *Definition of suicide.* New York: Wiley & Sons.

Simon, R. I. (1987). *Clinical psychiatry and the law.* Washington, DC: American Psychiatric Press.

Takahashi, Y. (1989). Suicidal Asian patients: Recommendations for treatment. *Suicide and Life-Threatening Behavior, 19,* 305-313.

Takahashi, Y. (1992). *Clinical evaluation of suicide risk and crisis intervention.* Tokyo: Kongoshuppan (in Japanese).

Takahashi, Y. (1993a). Suicide prevention in Japan. In A. A. Leenaars (Ed.), *Suicidology: Essays in honor of Edwin S. Shneidman* (pp. 324-334). Northvale, NJ: Jason Aronson.

Takahashi, Y. (1993b). Depression and suicide. In T. Kariya & M. Nakagawara (Eds.), *Affective disorders: Perspectives on basic research and clinical practice* (pp. 85-98). New York: Brunner/Mazel.

Takahashi, Y. (1995). Recent trends in suicidal behavior in Japan. *Psychiatry and Clinical Neurosciences, 49*(Suppl. 1), S105-S109.

Takahashi, Y., Hirasawa, H., Koyama, K., Asakawa, O., Kido, M., Onose, H., Udagawa, M., Ishikawa, Y., & Uno, M. (1995). Suicide and aging in Japan: An examination of treated elderly attempters. *International Psychogeriatrics, 7,* 239-251.

Suicide and Life-Threatening Behavior, Vol. 27, No. 1, Spring 1997

Index